D0827851

A FEAST OF INFORMATION—
for people who love to eat but need to know the carbohydrate count of their meals.

THE BARBARA KRAUS 1985 CARBOHYDRATE GUIDE TO BRAND NAMES & BASIC FOODS lists thousands of basic and ready-to-eat foods from appetizers to desserts—carry it to the supermarket, to the restaurant, to the beach, to the coffee cart, and on trips.

Flip through these fact-filled pages. Mix, match, and keep track of your carbohydrate intake.

The Barbara Kraus 1985 Carbohydrate Guide to Brand Names and Basic Foods

SIGNET Books by Barbara Kraus

(0451)

☐ **CALORIES AND CARBOHYDRATES by Barbara Kraus. Revised edition.** This complete guide contains over 8,000 brand names and basic foods with their caloric and carbohydrate counts. Recommended by doctors, nutritionists, and family food planners as an indispensable aid to those who must be concerned with what they eat, it will become the most important diet reference source you will ever own. (123301—$3.95)*

☐ **THE BARBARA KRAUS CALORIE GUIDE TO BRAND NAMES & BASIC FOODS, 1984 Edition.** Count calories with this—the most up-to-date and accurate calorie counter that lists thousands of basic and ready-to-eat foods from appetizers to desserts. (126912—$1.95)*

☐ **THE BARBARA KRAUS CARBOHYDRATE GUIDE TO BRAND NAMES & BASIC FOODS, 1984 Edition.** At a glance you'll know the carbohydrate count of many of your favorite brand name and basic foods, with this, the most up-to-date, accurate carbohydrate counter. (126920—$1.95)*

☐ **THE BARBARA KRAUS SODIUM GUIDE TO BRAND NAME & BASIC FOODS, 1984 Edition.** This complete guide contains a feast of information for people who love to eat but need to know the sodium count of their meals. (126939—$1.95)*

☐ **THE BARBARA KRAUS DICTIONARY OF PROTEIN.** The most complete and accurate listing published of the protein and caloric count per individual serving of thousands of brand names and basic foods. (087917—$2.50)

*Prices slightly higher in Canada

Buy them at your local bookstore or use this convenient coupon for ordering.
NEW AMERICAN LIBRARY,
P.O. Box 999, Bergenfield, New Jersey 07621
Please send me the books I have checked above. I am enclosing $________
(please add $1.00 to this order to cover postage and handling). Send check or money order—no cash or C.O.D.'s. Prices and numbers are subject to change without notice.
Name ________________
Address ________________
City ________ State ________ Zip Code ________
Allow 4-6 weeks for delivery.
This offer is subject to withdrawal without notice.

The Barbara Kraus 1985 Carbohydrate Guide to Brand Names and Basic Foods

A SIGNET BOOK
NEW AMERICAN LIBRARY

NAL BOOKS ARE AVAILABLE AT QUANTITY DISCOUNTS
WHEN USED TO PROMOTE PRODUCTS OR SERVICES.
FOR INFORMATION PLEASE WRITE TO PREMIUM MARKETING DIVISION,
NEW AMERICAN LIBRARY, 1633 BROADWAY,
NEW YORK, NEW YORK 10019.

Copyright © 1971, 1973, 1975, 1976, 1977 by Barbara Kraus.
© 1978 by John R. Fernbach, Esq. and Murray Cohen,
Co-Executors to the Estate of Barbara Kraus.
Copyright © 1979, 1980, 1981, 1982, 1983, 1984 by New American Library,

All rights reserved.

Excerpted from *Dictionary of Calories and Carbohydrates*

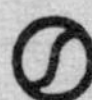

SIGNET TRADEMARK REG. U.S. PAT. OFF. AND FOREIGN COUNTRIES
REGISTERED TRADEMARK—MARCA REGISTRADA
HECHO EN CHICAGO, U.S.A.

SIGNET, SIGNET CLASSIC, MENTOR, PLUME, MERIDIAN AND NAL BOOKS
are published by New American Library,
1633 Broadway, New York, New York 10019

FIRST PRINTING, JANUARY, 1985

1 2 3 4 5 6 7 8 9

PRINTED IN THE UNITED STATES OF AMERICA

For Nick, Eileen
and Nicholas Romaniello

Foreword

The composition of the foods we eat is not static: it changes from time to time. In the case of *brand-name* products, manufacturers alter their recipes to reflect the availability of ingredients, advances in technology, or improvements in formulae. Each year new products appear on the market and some old ones are discontinued.

On the other hand, information on *basic foods* such as meats, vegetables, and fruits may also change as a result of the development of better analytical methods, different growing conditions, or new marketing practices. These changes, however, are usually relatively small as compared with those in manufactured products.

Some differences may be found between the values in this book and those appearing on the product labels. This is usually due to the fact that the Food and Drug Administration permits manufacturers to round the figures reported on labels. The data in this book are reported as calculated without rounding. If large differences between the two sets of values are noted, they may be due to changes in product formulae, and in those cases the label data should be used.

For all these reasons, a book of carbohydrate or nutritive values of foods must be kept up to date by a periodic reviewing and revision of the data presented.

Therefore, this handy carbohydrate counter will provide each year the most current and accurate estimates available. Generous use of this little book will help you and your family to select the right foods and the proper number of carbohydrates each member requires.

Good eating in 1985! For 1986, we'll pick up the new products, drop any has-beens, and make whatever other changes are necessary.

Barbara Kraus

Why This Book?

Some of the data presented here can be found in more detail in my best-selling *Calories and Carbohydrates,* a dictionary of 8,000 brand names and basic foods. Complete as it is, it is meant to be used as a reference book at home or in the office and not to be squeezed into a suit jacket or evening bag—it's just too big.

Therefore, responding to the need for a portable carbohydrate guide, and one which can reflect food changes often, I have written this smaller and handier version. The selection of material and the additional new entries provide readers with pertinent data on thousands of products that they can prepare at home to take to work, eat in a restaurant or luncheonette, nibble on from the coffee cart, take to the beach, buy in the candy store, etcetera.

For the sake of saving space and providing you with a greater selection of products, I had to make certain compromises: whereas in the giant book there are several physical descriptions of a product, here there is but one.

What Are Carbohydrates?

Carbohydrates—which include sugars, starches, and acids—are one of several chemical compounds in food which yield calories. Their main function is to supply energy to body cells, particularly muscle and brain cells. The amount of carbohydrates varies from zero in meats, fish, and poultry, to heavy concentrations in such foods as syrups, cereals, bread, beans, some fresh and all dried fruit, and root vegetables, such as potatoes.

As of this date, the most respected nutritional researchers insist that some carbohydrate is necessary every day for maintaining good health. The amount to be included is an individual matter, and in any drastic effort to alter your eating patterns, be sure to consult your doctor first.

ABBREVIATIONS AND SYMBOLS

* = prepared as package directs[1]
< = less than
& = and
" = inch
canned = bottles or jars as well as cans
dia. = diameter
fl. = fluid
liq. = liquid
lb. = pound
med. = medium
oz. = ounce
pkg. = package
pt. = pint
qt. = quart
sq. = square
T. = tablespoon
Tr. = trace
tsp. = teaspoon
wt. = weight

Italics or name in parentheses = registered trademark, ®. All data not identified by company or trademark are based on material obtained from the United States Department of Agriculture or Health, Education and Welfare/Food and Agriculture Organization.

EQUIVALENTS

By Weight
1 pound = 16 ounces
1 ounce = 28.35 grams
3.52 ounces = 100 grams

By Volume
1 quart = 4 cups
1 cup = 8 fluid ounces
1 cup = ½ pint
1 cup = 16 tablespoons
2 tablespoons = 1 fluid ounce
1 tablespoon = 3 teaspoons
1 pound butter = 4 sticks or 2 cups

[1]If the package directions call for whole or skim milk, the data given here are for whole milk unless otherwise stated.

A

Food and Description	*Measure or Quantity*	*Carbohydrates (grams)*
ABALONE, canned	4 oz.	2.6
AC'CENT	¼ tsp.	0.
ALBACORE, raw, meat only	4 oz.	0.
ALEXANDER COCKTAIL MIX		
(Holland House)	1 serving	16.0
ALLSPICE (French's)	1 tsp.	1.3
ALMOND:		
In shell	10 nuts	2.0
Shelled, raw, natural, with skins	1 oz.	5.5
Roasted, dry (Planters)	1 oz.	6.0
Roasted, oil (Fisher)	1 oz.	5.5
ALMOND EXTRACT		
(Virginia Dare) 34% alcohol	1 tsp.	0.
ALPHA-BITS**,** cereal (Post)	1 cup (1 oz.)	24.6
AMARETTO DI SARONNO	1 fl. oz.	9.0
A.M. FRUIT DRINK	6 fl. oz.	22.0
ANCHOVY, PICKLED, canned, flat or rolled, not heavily salted, drained	2-oz. can	.1
ANISE SEED, dried	½ oz.	6.3
ANISETTE:		
(DeKuyper)	1 fl. oz.	11.4
(Mr. Boston)	1 fl. oz.	10.8
APPLE:		
Eaten with skin	2½" dia.	15.3
Eaten without skin	2½" dia.	13.9
Canned (Comstock):		
Rings, drained	1 ring	7.0
Sliced	⅙ of 21-oz. can	10.0
Dried:		
(Del Monte)	2-oz. serving	37.0
(Sun-Maid/Sunsweet)	2-oz. serving	42.0
APPLE BROWN BETTY	1 cup	63.9
APPLE BUTTER (Smucker's) cider	1 T.	9.0

Food and Description	*Measure or Quantity*	*Carbohydrates (grams)*
APPLE-CHERRY JUICE,		
COCKTAIL,		
canned, *Musselman's*	8 fl. oz.	28.0
APPLE CIDER:		
Canned (Mott's) sweet	½ cup	14.6
*Mix, *Country Time*	8 fl. oz.	24.5
APPLE-CRANBERRY DRINK		
(Hi-C):		
Canned	6 fl. oz.	21.0
*Mix	6 fl. oz.	18.0
APPLE-CRANBERRY JUICE,		
canned (Lincoln)	6 fl. oz.	25.0
APPLE DRINK:		
Canned:		
Capri Sun, natural	6¾ fl. oz.	22.7
(Hi-C)	6 fl. oz.	23.0
*Mix (Hi-C)	6 fl. oz.	18.0
APPLE DUMPLINGS, frozen		
(Pepperidge Farm)	1 dumpling	33.0
APPLE, ESCALLOPED, frozen		
(Stouffer's)	4 oz.	28.0
APPLE-GRAPE JUICE, canned:		
Musselman's	6 fl. oz.	21.0
(Red Cheek)	6 fl. oz.	22.6
APPLE JACKS, cereal (Kellogg's)	1 cup (1 oz.)	26.0
APPLE JAM (Smucker's)	1 T.	13.5
APPLE JELLY:		
Sweetened (Smucker's)	1 T.	14.0
Dietetic:		
(Dia-Mel; Louis Sherry)	1 T.	0.
(Diet Delight)	1 T.	3.0
(Featherweight)	1 T.	4.0
APPLE JUICE:		
Canned:		
(Lincoln)	6 fl. oz.	24.0
(Mott's)	6 fl. oz.	19.0
Musselman's	6 fl. oz.	21.0
(Ocean Spray)	6 fl. oz.	23.0
(Red Cheek)	6 fl. oz.	21.2
Chilled (Minute Maid)	6 fl. oz.	24.0
*Frozen:		
(Minute Maid)	6 fl. oz.	24.0
(Seneca Foods)	6 fl. oz.	22.0
APPLE PIE (See PIE, Apple)		
APPLE SAUCE:		
Regular:		

Food and Description	*Measure or Quantity*	*Carbohydrates (grams)*
(Del Monte)	½ cup	24.0
(Mott's) natural style or with ground cranberries	½ cup	27.5
Musselman's	½ cup	23.5
Dietetic:		
(Del Monte) Lite	½ cup	13.0
(Diet Delight)	½ cup	13.0
(Mott's)	½ cup	11.0
(S&W) *Nutradiet*	½ cup	14.0
APPLE STRUDEL, frozen (Pepperidge Farm)	3 oz.	35.0
APRICOT:		
Fresh, whole	1 apricot	4.6
Canned, regular pack:		
(Del Monte) whole, peeled	½ cup	27.0
(Stokely-Van Camp)	1 cup	54.0
Canned, dietetic:		
(Del Monte) Lite	½ cup	16.0
(Diet Delight):		
Syrup pack	½ cup	15.0
Water pack	½ cup	9.0
(Featherweight):		
Juice pack	½ cup	12.0
Water pack	½ cup	9.0
(S&W) *Nutradiet:*		
Halves, white or blue label	½ cup	9.0
Whole, juice	½ cup	7.0
Dried:		
(Del Monte)	2 oz.	35.0
(Sun-Maid/Sunsweet)	2 oz.	35.0
APRICOT LIQUEUR (DeKuyper)	1 fl. oz.	8.3
APRICOT NECTAR (Del Monte)	6 fl. oz.	26.0
APRICOT-PINEAPPLE NECTAR, canned, dietetic (S&W) *Nutradiet,* blue label	6 oz.	12.0
APRICOT & PINEAPPLE PRESERVE OR JAM:		
Sweetened (Smucker's)	1 T.	13.5
Deitetic:		
(Diet Delight)	1 T.	3.0
(Featherweight)	1 T.	1.0
APRICOT PRESERVES, dietetic (Louis Sherry)	1 T.	0.
APRICOT SOUR COCKTAIL (National Distillers) *Duet* 12½% alcohol	2 fl. oz.	1.6

Food and Description	*Measure or Quantity*	*Carbohydrates (grams)*
ARBY'S:		
Bac'n Cheddar Deluxe	1 sandwich	35.0
Beef & Cheddar Sandwich	6 oz.	46.0
Chicken Breast Sandwich	1 sandwich	55.0
French dip	1 sandwich	47.0
Ham 'N Cheese	1 sandwich	46.0
Potato cakes	2 pieces	24.0
Roast Beef:		
Regular	5 oz.	32.0
Deluxe	1 sandwich	43.0
Junior	1 sandwich	21.0
Super	1 sandwich	61.0
Sauce:		
Arby's	1 oz.	7.0
Horsey	1 oz.	5.0
ARTICHOKE:		
Boiled	15-oz. artichoke	42.1
Canned (Cara Mia) marinated, drained	6-oz. jar	12.6
Frozen (Birds Eye) deluxe, hearts	⅓ pkg.	6.6
ASPARAGUS:		
Boiled	1 spear (½" dia. at base)	.5
Canned, regular pack, spears, solid & liq.:		
(Del Monte) green or white	4 oz.	3.0
(Green Giant) green	4 oz.	3.2
(Le Sueur)	4 oz.	4.0
Canned, dietetic, solids & liq.:		
(Diet Delight)	½ cup	2.0
(S&W) *Nutradiet*, green label	½ cup	3.0
Frozen:		
(Birds Eye);		
Cuts	⅓ pkg.	3.8
Spears, regular or jumbo deluxe	⅓ pkg.	3.9
(Green Giant) cuts, butter sauce	3 oz.	6.0
(Stouffer's) souffle	⅓ pkg.	8.0
AUNT JEMIMA SYRUP (See SYRUP)		
AVOCADO, all varities	1 fruit (10.7 oz.)	14.3
****AWAKE*** (Birds Eye)	6 fl. oz.	20.5
AYDS:		
Butterscotch	1 piece	5.7
Chocolate, chocolate mint, vanilla	1 piece	5.5

B

Food and Description	Measure or Quantity	Carbohydrates (grams)
BACON, cooked:		
(Oscar Mayer):		
Regular slice	6-gram slice	.1
Thick slice	1 slice	.2
Range Brand (Hormel)	1 slice	0.
BACON BITS:		
*Bac*Os* (Betty Crocker)	1 tsp.	.7
(Durkee) imitation	1 tsp.	.5
(French's) imitation	1 tsp.	Tr.
(Hormel)	1 tsp.	0.
(McCormick) imitation	1 tsp.	.7
(Oscar Mayer) real	1 tsp.	.1
BACON, CANADIAN, unheated:		
(Eckrich)	1 oz.	1.0
(Hormel) sliced	1 oz.	0.
(Oscar Mayer) 93% fat free	1-oz. slice	0.
BACON, SIMULATED, cooked:		
(Oscar Mayer) *Lean 'N Tasty*, beef or pork	1 slice	.2
(Swift's) *Sizzlean*	1 strip	0.
BAGEL:		
Egg	3 inch dia. (1.9 oz.)	28.3
Water	3 inch dia. (1.9 oz.)	30.5
BAKING POWDER:		
(Calumet)	1 tsp.	.6
(Featherweight) low sodium, cereal free	1 tsp.	2.0
BAMBOO SHOOTS:		
Raw, trimmed	¼ lb.	5.9
Canned, drained (La Choy)	¼ cup	1.0
BANANA, medium (Dole)	6-oz. banana (weighed unpeeled)	26.4
BANANA NECTAR (Libby's)	6 fl. oz.	14.0

Food and Description	*Measure or Quantity*	*Carbohydrates (grams)*
BANANA PIE (See PIE, Banana)		
BARBECUE SEASONING		
(French's)	1 tsp.	1.0
BARBERA WINE		
(Louis M. Martini)	3 fl. oz.	.2
BARDOLINO WINE (Antinori)	1 fl. oz.	6.3
BARLEY, pearled (Quaker Scotch)	¼ cup	36.3
BASIL (French's)	1 tsp.	.7
BASS	any quantity	0.
BAY LEAF (French's)	1 tsp.	1.0
B & B LIQUEUR	1 fl. oz.	5.7
B.B.Q. SAUCE & BEEF, frozen		
(Banquet) *Cookin' Bag,* sliced	4-oz. pkg.	13.0
BEAN, BAKED:		
(USDA):		
With pork & molasses sauce	1 cup	53.8
With pork & tomato sauce	1 cup	48.5
Canned:		
(B&M) *Brick Oven*	8-oz. serving	50.0
(Campbell):		
Home style	8-oz. can	48.0
With pork & tomato sauce	8-oz. can	49.0
(Friend's) red kidney	9-oz. serving	56.3
(Grandma Brown's)	8-oz.	54.1
(Howard Johnson's)	1 cup	21.1
(Libby's) *Deep Brown*	¼ of 14-oz. can	40.6
(Van Camp) with pork	8 oz.	41.3
BEAN, BARBECUE (Campbell)	7⅞-oz. can	43.0
BEAN, BLACK OR BROWN, DRY	1 cup	122.4
BEAN & FRANKFURTER, canned:		
(Campbell) in tomato and molasses sauce	7⅞-oz. can	42.0
(Hormel) *Short Orders,* 'n wieners	7½-oz. can	29.0
BEAN & FRANKFURTER DINNER, frozen:		
(Banquet)	10¼-oz. dinner	64.0
(Morton)	10¾-oz. dinner	79.0
BEAN, GARBANZO, canned, dietetic (S&W) *Nutradiet,* low sodium, green label	½ cup	19.0
BEAN, GREEN:		
Boiled, 1½" to 2" pieces, drained	½ cup	3.7
Canned, regular pack, solids & liq.:		
(Comstock)	½ cup	4.0
(Del Monte) French	½ cup	4.0
(Green Giant) French or whole	½ cup	4.2

Food and Description	*Measure or Quantity*	*Carbohydrates (grams)*
(Libby's) French	½ cup	2.7
(Sunshine)	½ cup	3.8
Canned, dietetic, solids & liq.:		
(Del Monte) no salt added	4 oz.	4.0
(Diet Delight)	½ cup	3.0
(Featherweight)	½ cup	5.0
(S&W) *Nutradiet*, cut	½ cup	4.0
Frozen:		
(Birds Eye);		
Cut or French	⅓ pkg.	5.9
French, with almonds	⅓ pkg.	8.4
Whole, deluxe	⅓ pkg.	5.1
(Green Giant):		
With butter sauce	½ cup	6.0
With mushroom in cream sauce	½ cup	10.0
Polybag	½ cup	4.0
(McKenzie) cut or French style	⅓ pkg.	6.0
BEAN, GREEN & MUSHROOM, CASSEROLE (Stouffer's)	½ pkg.	12.0
BEAN, GREEN, WITH POTATOES, canned (Sunshine) solids & liq.	½ cup	7.0
BEAN, ITALIAN:		
Canned (Del Monte) solids & liq.	½ cup	6.0
Frozen (McKenzie, Seabrook Farms)	⅓ pkg.	7.1
BEAN, KIDNEY:		
Canned, regular pack, solids & liq.:		
(Furman) red, fancy, light	½ cup	21.2
(Van Camp):		
Light	8 oz.	35.9
New Orleans style	8 oz.	33.8
Red	8 oz.	37.9
Canned, dietetic (S&W) *Nutradiet*, low sodium, green label, solids & liq.	½ cup	16.0
BEAN, LIMA:		
Boiled, drained	½ cup	16.8
Canned, regular pack, solids & liq.:		
(Del Monte)	½ cup	14.0
(Libby's)	½ cup	16.0
Canned, dietetic (Featherweight) solids & liq.	½ cup	16.0
Frozen:		
(Birds Eye), tiny, deluxe	⅓ pkg.	20.3
(Green Giant);		

Food and Description	*Measure or Quantity*	*Carbohydrates (grams)*
In butter sauce	½ cup	20.0
Harvest Fresh	½ cup	19.0
(McKenzie) Fordhook	⅓ pkg.	19.0
(Seabrook Farms):		
Baby butter bean	⅓ pkg.	26.1
Fordhooks	⅓ pkg.	17.9
BEAN, PINTO:		
Canned (Del Monte)	½ cup	19.0
Frozen (McKenzie)	3.2 oz.	29.0
BEAN, REFRIED, canned:		
(Del Monte) regular or spicy	½ cup	20.0
Old El Paso:		
Plain	4 oz.	17.0
With sausage	4 oz.	14.8
(Ortega) lightly spicy or true bean	½ cup	25.0
BEAN SALAD, canned:		
(Green Giant)	4¼-oz. serving	18.0
(Nalley's)	4½-oz. serving	29.4
BEAN SOUP (See SOUP, Bean)		
BEAN SPROUT:		
Mung, raw	½ lb.	15.0
Mung, boiled, drained	¼ lb.	5.9
Soy, raw	½ lb.	12.0
Soy, boiled, drained	¼ lb.	4.2
Canned (La Choy) drained	⅔ cup	1.0
BEAN, YELLOW OR WAX:		
Boiled, 1" pieces, drained	½ cup	3.7
Canned, regular pack, solids & liq.:		
(Comstock)	½ cup	4.5
(Del Monte)	½ cup	4.0
(Libby's) cut	4 oz.	4.4
Canned, dietetic (Featherweight) cut, solids & liq.	½ cup	5.0
Frozen (McKenzie) cut	⅓ pkg.	5.0
BEEF	Any quantity	0.
BEEF BOUILLON:		
(Herb-Ox):		
Cube	1 cube	.7
Packet	1 packet	.9
MBT	1 packet	2.0
Low sodium (Featherweight)	1 tsp.	2.0
BEEF, CHIPPED, CREAMED:		
Cooked, home recipe	½ cup	8.7
Frozen, creamed		
(Banquet) *Cookin' Bag*	4-oz. pkg.	8.0
(Morton)	5-oz. pkg.	9.0

Food and Description	*Measure or Quantity*	*Carbohydrates (grams)*
(Stouffer's)	5½-oz. serving	10.0
(Swanson)	10½-oz. entree	16.0
BEEF DINNER or ENTREE, frozen:		
(Banquet):		
American Favorites, chopped	11-oz. dinner	23.0
Extra Helping, sliced	16-oz. dinner	72.0
(Green Giant) baked, teriyaki	10-oz. entree	36.0
(Morton):		
Regular	10-oz. dinner	20.0
Country Table, sliced	14-oz. dinner	57.0
Steak House, sirloin strip	9½-oz. dinner	43.0
(Stouffer's) *Lean Cuisine*, oriental	8⅝-oz. dinner	32.0
(Swanson):		
Hungry Man:		
Chopped	18-oz. dinner	50.0
Sliced	12¼-oz. entree	20.0
TV Brand, chopped sirloin	10-oz. dinner	33.0
3-course	15-oz. dinner	50.0
(Weight Watchers):		
Beefsteak, 2-compartment meal	9¾-oz. pkg.	14.0
Oriental	10-oz. pkg.	32.1
Sirloin in mushroom sauce, 3-compartment meal	13-oz. pkg.	16.0
BEEF, DRIED, canned (Hormel) *Short Orders*, creamed	7½-oz. can	9.0
BEEF GOULASH (Hormel) *Short Orders*	7½-oz. can	17.0
BEEF, GROUND, SEASONING MIX:		
*(Durkee):		
Regular	1 cup	9.0
With onion	1 cup	6.5
(French's) with onion	1⅛-oz. pkg.	24.0
BEEF HASH, ROAST:		
Canned, *Mary Kitchen* (Hormel) regular or *Short Orders*	7½-oz. serving	18.0
Frozen (Stouffer's)	½ of 11½-oz. can	11.0
BEEF, PACKAGED (Hormel)	1-oz. serving	0.
BEEF PEPPER ORIENTAL: frozen (La Choy):		
Dinner	12-oz. dinner	45.0
Entree	12-oz. entree	18.0
BEEF PIE, frozen:		
(Banquet):		
Regular	8-oz. pie	47.0
Supreme	8-oz. pie	38.0

Food and Description	*Measure or Quantity*	*Carbohydrates (grams)*
(Morton)	8-oz. pie	31.0
(Stouffer's)	10-oz. pie	38.0
(Swanson) *Hungry Man*	16-oz. pie	65.0
BEEF PUFFS, frozen (Durkee)	1 piece	3.0
BEEF, SHORT RIBS, frozen		
(Stouffer's) boneless, with vegetable gravy	½ of 11½-oz. pkg.	2.0
BEEF SOUP (See SOUP, Beef)		
BEEF SPREAD, ROAST, canned		
(Underwood)	½ of 4¾-oz. can	Tr.
BEEF STEAK, BREADED, frozen		
(Hormel)	4-oz. serving	13.9
BEEF STEW:		
Home recipe, made with lean beef chuck	1 cup	15.2
Canned, regular pack:		
Dinty Moore (Hormel):		
Regular	8-oz. serving	15.0
Short Orders	7½-oz. can	14.0
(Libby's)	7½-oz. serving	18.0
(Swanson)	7⅝-oz. serving	16.0
Canned, dietetic:		
(Dia-Mel)	8-oz. serving	19.0
(Featherweight)	7½-oz. serving	24.0
Frozen:		
(Banquet) *Buffet Supper*	2-lb. pkg.	84.0
(Green Giant), *Boil 'N Bag*	9-oz. entree	20.0
(Morton) *Family Meal*	2-lb. pkg.	56.0
(Stouffer's)	10-oz. serving	16.0
BEEF STEW SEASONING MIX:		
*(Durkee)	1 cup.	16.7
(French's)	1 pkg.	30.0
BEEF STOCK BASE (French's)	1 tsp.	2.0
BEEF STROGANOFF, frozen		
(Stouffer's) with parsley noodles	9¾ oz.	31.0
***BEEF STROGANOFF SEASONING MIX** (Durkee)	1 cup	71.2
BEER & ALE:		
Regular:		
Black Horse Ale	8 fl. oz.	8.9
Budweiser	8 fl. oz.	9.1
Busch Bavarian	8 fl. oz.	9.0
Michelob	8 fl. oz.	9.0
Light or low carbohydrate:		
Budweiser Light	8 fl. oz.	4.5
Michelob Light	8 fl. oz.	7.8

Food and Description	*Measure or Quantity*	*Carbohydrates (grams)*
Natural Light	8 fl. oz.	4.0
Stroh Light	8 fl. oz.	4.7
BEER, NEAR:		
Goetz Pale	8 fl. oz.	2.6
Kingsbury (Heileman)	8 fl. oz.	7.6
BEET:		
Boiled, whole	2" dia. beet	3.6
Boiled, sliced	½ cup	7.3
Canneds, regular pack solids & liq.:		
(Del Monte)		
Pickled	4 oz.	19.0
Sliced or whole	4 oz.	8.0
(Greenwood) pickled	½ cup	27.5
(Libby's) Harvard	½ cup	20.8
(Stokely-Van Camp) pickled	½ cup	22.5
Canned, dietetic, solids & liq.:		
(Comstock)	½ cup	6.5
(Del Monte) No Salt Added	½ cup	8.0
(Featherweight) sliced	½ cup	10.0
(S&W) *Nutradiet*, sliced, green label	½ cup	9.0
BENEDICTINE LIQUEUR (Julius Wile)	1 fl. oz.	10.3
BIG H, burger sauce (Hellmann's)	1 T.	1.6
BIG MAC (See *McDONALD'S*)		
BIG WHEELS (Hostess)	1 piece	21.0
BISCUIT DOUGH (Pillsbury):		
Baking Powder, *1869 Brand*	1 biscuit	13.5
Big Country	1 biscuit	15.5
Buttermilk:		
Regular	1 biscuit	10.0
Extra Lights	1 biscuit	10.5
Butter Tastin', 1869 Brand	1 biscuit	11.0
Dinner	1 biscuit	7.5
Oven Ready, Ballard	1 biscuit	9.5
BLACKBERRY, fresh, hulled	1 cup	18.8
BLACKBERRY JELLY:		
Sweetened (Smucker's)	1 T.	13.5
Dietetic:		
(Dia-Mel)	1 T.	3.0
(Featherweight)	1 T.	4.0
BLACKBERRY LIQUEUR (Bols)	1 fl. oz.	8.9
BLACKBERRY PRESERVE OR JAM:		
Sweetened (Smucker's)	1 T.	13.5

Food and Description	Measure or Quantity	Carbohydrates (grams)
Dietetic:		
(Dia-Mel; Louis Sherry)	1 T.	0.
(Diet-Delight)	1 T.	3.3
(Featherweight)	1 T.	4.0
(S&W) *Nutradiet*	1 T.	3.0
BLACKBERRY WINE		
(Mogen David)	3 fl. oz.	18.7
BLACK-EYED PEAS:		
Canned, with pork, solids & liq.		
(Sunshine)	½ cup	16.1
Frozen:		
(Birds Eye)	⅓ of pkg.	23.5
(McKenzie)	⅓ pkg.	23.0
(Southland)	⅓ of 16-oz. pkg.	21.0
BLINTZE, frozen (King Kold) cheese	2½-oz. piece	21.4
Dry (Bar-Tender's)	1 serving	5.7
Liquid (Sacramento)	5½-fl.-oz. can	9.1
BLUEBERRY, fresh, trimmed	½ cup	11.2
BLUEBERRY PIE (See PIE, Blueberry)		
BLUEBERRY PRESERVE OR JAM:		
Sweetened (Smucker's)	1 T.	13.5
Dietetic (Dia-Mel; Louis Sherry)	1 T.	0.
BLUEFISH, broiled	3½" × 3" × ½" piece	0.
BODY BUDDIES, cereal		
(General Mills) brown sugar & honey or natural fruit flavor	1 cup	24.0
BOLOGNA:		
(Eckrich):		
Beef	1-oz. slice	2.0
Beef, thick slice	1.8-oz. slice	3.0
Beef, thin slice	1 slice	1.0
Garlic	1-oz. slice	2.0
Meat, regular slice	1-oz. slice	2.0
Meat, thick slice	1.7-oz. slice	3.0
Sandwich	1-oz. slice	2.0
(Hormel):		
Beef	1-oz. serving	.5
Meat	1-oz. slice	0.
(Oscar Mayer):		
Beef	.8-oz. slice	.6
Beef	1-oz. slice	.8
Beef	1.3-oz. slice	1.1
Meat	.8-oz. slice	.4
Meat	1-oz. slice	.5
(Swift)	1-oz. slice	1.5

Food and Description	*Measure or Quantity*	*Carbohydrates (grams)*
BOLOGNA & CHEESE:		
(Eckrich)	.7-oz slice	2.0
(Oscar Mayer)	.8-oz. slice	.6
BONITO, canned	Any quantity	0.
BOO*BERRY, cereal (General Mills)	1 cup	24.0
BORSCHT, canned:		
Regular:		
(Gold's)	8-oz. serving	17.5
(Mother's) old fashioned	8-oz. serving	21.3
Dietetic or low calorie		
(Gold's)	8-oz. serving	17.5
(Mother's):		
Artificially sweetened	8-oz. serving	6.1
Unsalted	8-oz. serving	25.1
(Rokeach)	8-oz. serving	6.7
BOSCO (see SYRUP)		
BOYSENBERRY JELLY:		
Sweetened (Smucker's)	1 T.	13.5
Dietetic (S&W) *Nutradiet*	1 T.	3.0
BRAN:		
Crude	1 oz.	17.5
Miller's (Elam's)	1 oz.	13.7
BRAN BREAKFAST CEREAL:		
(Crawford's) dates	⅓ cup	20.0
(Kellogg's):		
All Bran or *Bran Buds*	⅓ cup	22.0
Cracklin' Oat Bran	½ cup	20.0
Raisin	¾ cup	30.0
(Nabisco)	½ cup	21.0
(Post) 40% bran flakes	⅔ cup	22.5
(Quaker) *Corn Bran*	⅔ cup	23.3
(Ralston-Purina):		
Bran Chex or 40% bran	⅔ cup	23.0
Honey	⅞ cup	24.0
Raisin	¾ cup	30.0
BRANDY, FLAVORED		
(Mr. Boston):		
Apricot or peach	1 fl. oz.	8.9
Blackberry	1 fl. oz.	8.6
Cherry	1 fl. oz.	7.4
BRAUNSCHWEIGER (Eckrich; Oscar Mayer) chub	1 oz.	1.0
BRAZIL NUT:		
Shelled	4 nuts	1.9
Roasted (Fisher) salted	1 oz.	3.1

Food and Description	Measure or Quantity	Carbohydrates (grams)
BREAD:		
Apple (Pepperidge Farm)		
with cinnamon	.9-oz. slice	13.0
Boston Brown	3″ × ¾″ slice	21.9
Bran (Arnold)		
Bran 'rola	1.2-oz. slice	15.5
Cinnamon (Pepperidge Farm)	.9-oz. slice	12.5
Corn & Molasses		
(Pepperidge Farm)	.9-oz. slice	15.0
Cracked wheat:		
(Pepperidge Farm)	.9-oz. slice	13.0
(Wonder)	1-oz. slice	13.0
Crispbrad, *Wasa:*		
Mora	3.-2oz. slice	70.5
Rye, golden	.4-oz. slice	7.8
Rye, lite	.3-oz. slice	6.2
Sesame	.5-oz. slice	10.6
Date nut roll (Dromedary)	1-oz. slice	13.0
Date walnut (Pepperidge Farm)	.9-oz. slice	11.5
Flatbread, *Ideal:*		
Bran	.2-oz. slice	4.1
Extra thin	.1-oz. slice	2.5
Whole grain	.2-oz. slice	4.0
French:		
(Arnold) Vienna	1-oz. slice	14.5
(Pepperidge Farm) fully baked	2-oz. slice	28.0
(Wonder)	1-oz. slice	13.0
Hillbilly	1-oz. slice	14.0
Hollywood, dark	1-oz. slice	13.0
Honey bran (Pepperidge Farm)	1.2-oz. slice	13.0
Honey wheat berry (Arnold)	1.2-oz. slice	16.0
Italian (Pepperidge Farm)	2-oz. slice	27.0
Multi-grain (Pepperidge Farm)	.5-oz. slice	7.0
Oatmeal (Pepperidge Farm)	.9-oz. slice	12.5
Onion (Pepperidge Farm) party	.2-oz. slice	2.8
Orange & Raisin		
(Pepperidge Farm)	.9-oz. slice	12.5
Pumpernickel:		
(Arnold)	1-oz. slice	14.0
(Levy's)	1.1-oz. slice	15.5
(Pepperidge Farm):		
Regular	1.1-oz. slice	15.5
Party	.2-oz. slice	3.0
Raisin:		
(Arnold) tea	.9-oz. slice	13.0
(Pepperidge Farm)	1 slice	14.0

Food and Description	*Measure or Quantity*	*Carbohydrates (grams)*
(Sun-Maid)	1-oz. slice	14.5
Roman Meal	1-oz. slice	13.0
Rye:		
(Arnold) Jewish	1.1-oz. slice	14.0
(Levy's) Real	1-oz. slice	15.0
(Pepperidge Farm):		
Family	1.1-oz. slice	15.5
Party	.2-oz. slice	3.2
(Wonder)	1-oz. slice	13.0
Sahara (Thomas') wheat	1-oz. piece	13.7
7-Grain, *Home Pride*	1-oz. slice	13.0
Sourdough, *Di Carlo*	1-oz. slice	14.0
Vienna (Pepperidge Farm)	.9-oz. slice	13.5
Wheat (see also Cracked Wheat or Whole Wheat):		
(Arnold) *Bran'nola*	1.3-oz. slice	17.5
Fresh Horizons	1-oz. slice	10.0
Fresh & Natural	1-oz. slice	13.0
Home Pride	1-oz. slice	13.0
(Pepperidge Farm) sandwich	.8-oz. slice	10.0
(Wonder) family	1-oz. slice	13.0
Wheatberry, *Home Pride*, honey	1-oz. slice	12.0
Wheat Germ (Pepperidge Farm)	.9-oz. slice	12.5
White:		
(Arnold):		
Brick Oven	.8-oz. slice	11.0
Measure Up	.5-oz. slice	7.0
Home Pride	1-oz. slice	13.0
(Pepperidge Farm):		
Large loaf	.9-oz. slice	13.5
Sandwich	.8-oz. slice	11.5
Toasting	1.2-oz. slice	16.0
(Wonder) regular or buttermilk	1-oz. slice	13.0
Whole wheat:		
(Arnold) *Brick Oven*	.8-oz. slice	9.5
(Pepperidge Farm) thin slice	1 slice	12.0
(Thomas') 100%	.8-oz. slice	10.1
BREAD, CANNED, brown, plain or raisin (B&M)	½" slice	18.2
BREAD CRUMBS:		
(Contadina) seasoned	½ cup	40.6
(Pepperidge Farm) regular or herb seasoned	1 oz.	22.0
***BREAD DOUGH, FROZEN:**		
(Pepperidge Farm):		
Country rye or white	1/10 of loaf	13.5

Food and Description	*Measure or Quantity*	*Carbohydrates (grams)*
Stone ground wheat	1/10 of loaf	14.0
(Rich's):		
French or Italian	1/20 of loaf	11.0
Wheat	.5-oz. slice	10.5
White	.8-oz. slice	9.4
***BREAD DOUGH, REFRIGERATED:** (Pillsbury)		
Poppin' Fresh:		
Rye or white	1/16 of loaf	21.0
Wheat	1/16 of loaf	20.0
***BREAD MIX:** (Pillsbury)		
Applesauce spice	1/12 of loaf	28.0
Apricot nut or carrot nut	1/12 of loaf	27.0
Cherry nut or nut	1/12 of loaf	30.0
BREAD STICK, DOUGH, refrigerated (Pillsbury)		
Pipin' Hot	1 piece	18.0
***BREAKFAST DRINK** (Pillsbury)	1 pouch	38.0
BREAKFAST SQUARES		
(General Mills) all flavors	1 bar	22.5
BROCCOLI:		
Boiled, whole stalk (6.3 oz.)	1 stalk	8.1
Boiled, ½" pieces	½ cup	3.5
Frozen:		
(Birds Eye):		
With almonds & selected seasonings	⅓ pkg.	5.7
In cheese sauce	⅓ pkg	8.4
Chopped	⅓ pkg.	4.5
Spears, regular	⅓ pkg.	4.9
(Green Giant):		
Cuts, polybag	½ cup	2.0
Harvest Fresh	4 oz.	4.0
Spears in butter sauce	3⅓ oz.	5.0
(McKenzie) chopped or spears	⅓ pkg.	5.0
(Stouffer's) in cheese sauce	4½-oz. serving	8.0
BROTH & SEASONING:		
(George Washington)	1 packet	1.0
Maggi	1 T.	.1
BRUSSELS SPROUT:		
Boiled	3-4 sprouts	3.9
Frozen:		
(Birds Eye):		
Baby, with cheese sauce	⅓ pkg.	8.7
Baby, deluxe	⅓ pkg.	7.3
In butter sauce	⅓ pkg.	7.2

Food and Description	*Measure or Quantity*	*Carbohydrates (grams)*
(Green Giant):		
In butter sauce	½ pkg.	9.0
Halves in cheese sauce	½ pkg.	13.0
(McKenzie)	3⅓ oz.	7.0
BUCKWHEAT, cracked (Pocono)	1 oz.	19.4
BUC*WHEATS, cereal		
(General Mills)	1 oz. (¾ cup)	24.0
BULGUR, canned, seasoned	4 oz.	37.2
BULLWINKLE PUDDING STIX,		
Good Humor	1¾-fl. oz. bar	15.0
BURGER KING:		
Apple pie	3-oz. pie	32.0
Cheeseburger	1 burger	30.0
Cheeseburger, double meat	1 burger	32.0
Coca Cola	1 medium-sized drink	31.0
French fries	1 regular order	25.0
Hamburger	1 burger	29.0
Onion rings	1 regular order	29.0
Pepsi, diet	1 medium-sized drink	1.6
Shake, chocolate	1 shake	57.0
Whopper:		
Regular	1 burger	50.0
Regular, with cheese	1 burger	52.0
Double beef	1 burger	52.0
Double beef, with cheese	1 burger	54.0
Junior	1 burger	31.0
Junior with cheese	1 burger	32.0
BURGUNDY WINE:		
(Louis M. Martini)	3 fl. oz.	.2
(Paul Masson)	3 fl. oz.	2.2
(Taylor)	3 fl. oz.	3.3
BURGUNDY WINE, SPARKLING:		
(B&G)	3 fl. oz.	2.2
(Taylor)	3 fl. oz.	4.2
BURRITO:		
*Canned (Del Monte)	1 burrito	39.0
Frozen:		
(Hormel):		
Beef	1 burrito	31.0
Cheese	1 burrito	32.0
Hot chili	1 burrito	33.0
(Van de Kamp's) & guacamole sauce	6-oz. serving	40.0

Food and Description	*Measure or Quantity*	*Carbohydrates (grams)*
BURRITO FILLING MIX, canned		
(Del Monte)	½ cup	20.0
BUTTER:		
Regular:		
(Breakstone)	1 T.	Tr.
(Meadow Gold)	1 tsp.	0.
Whipped (Breakstone)	1 T.	Tr.
BUTTERSCOTCH MORSELS		
(Nestlé)	1 oz.	19.0

C

Food and Description	*Measure or Quantity*	*Carbohydrates (grams)*
CABBAGE:		
Boiled, without salt	½ cup (2.6 oz.)	3.1
Canned, solids & liq.:		
(Comstock) red	½ cup	13.0
(Greenwood) red	½ cup	13.0
Frozen (Green Giant) stuffed	½ of entree	19.0
CABERNET SAUVIGNON		
(Paul Masson)	1 fl. oz.	.2
CAFE COMFORT, 55 proof	1 fl. oz.	8.8
CAKE:		
Regular, non-frozen:		
Plain, home recipe, with butter, with boiled white icing	⅑ of 9″ square	70.5
Angel food, home recipe	1/12 of 8″ cake	24.1
Caramel, home recipe, with caramel icing	⅑ of 9″ square	50.2
Chocolate, home recipe, with chocolate icing, 2-layer	1½ of 9″ cake	55.2
Crumb (Hostess)	1¼-oz. cake	22.0
Fruit:		
Home recipe, dark	1/30 of 8″ loaf	9.0
Home recipe, made with butter	1/30 of 8″ loaf	8.6
(Holland Honey Cake) unsalted	1¼ of cake	19.0
Pound, home recipe, traditional, made with butter	3½″ × 3½″ slice	16.4
Raisin Date Loaf (Holland Honey Cake) low sodium	1¼ of 13-oz. cake	19.0
Sponge, home recipe	1/12 of 10″ cake	35.7
White, home recipe, made with butter, without icing, 2-layer	⅑ of 9″ wide, 3′ high cake	50.8
Yellow, home recipe, made with butter, without icing, 2-layer	1/19 of cake	56.3

Food and Description	Measure or Quantity	Carbohydrates (grams)
Frozen:		
Apple Walnut:		
(Pepperidge Farm) with cream cheese icing	⅛ of 11¾-oz. cake	18.0
(Sara Lee)	⅛ of 12½-oz. cake	21.6
Banana nut		
(Sara Lee)	⅛ of 13¾-oz. cake	26.5
Carrot:		
(Pepperidge Farm)	⅛ of 11¾-oz. cake	17.0
(Weight Watchers)	2⅝-oz. serving	26.1
Cheesecake:		
(Morton) *Great Little Desserts:*		
Cherry	6-oz. cake	47.0
Strawberry	6-oz. cake	50.0
(Rich's) Viennese	1/14 of 42-oz. cake	24.1
(Sara Lee):		
Blueberry, *For 2*	½ of 11.3-oz. cake	66.6
Cream cheese:		
Regular	⅓ of 10-oz. cake	29.9
Cherry	⅙ of 19-oz. cake	35.2
Strawberry, French	⅛ of 26-oz. cake	27.5
Chocolate:		
(Pepperidge Farm):		
Layer, fudge	1/10 of 17-oz. cake	23.0
Rich 'N Moist with chocolate icing	⅛ of 14¼-oz. cake	23.0
Supreme	¼ of 11-½-oz. cake	37.0
(Sara Lee):		
Regular	⅛ of 13¼-oz. cake	21.0
Layer 'N Cream	⅛ of 18-oz. cake	23.8
Coffee (Sara Lee):		
Almond ring	⅛ of 9½-oz. cake	16.8
Apple	⅛ of 15-oz. cake	24.1
Apple, *For 2*	½ of 9-oz. cake	58.1
Maple crunch ring	⅛ of 9¾-oz. cake	17.3
Pecan	⅛ of 11¼-oz. cake	19.1
Streusel, butter	⅛ of 11½-oz. cake	20.3
Struesel, cinnamon	⅛ of 10.9-oz. cake	19.0
Crumb (See ROLL OR BUN, Crumb)		
Devil's Food (Pepperidge Farm) layer	1/10 of 17-oz. cake	24.0
Golden (Pepperidge Farm) layer	1/10 of 17-oz. cake	24.0
Lemon coconut		
(Pepperidge Farm)	¼ of 12¼-oz. cake	38.0
Orange (Sara Lee)	⅛ of 13¾-oz. cake	25.3

Food and Description	Measure or Quantity	Carbohydrates (grams)
Pineapple cream		
(Pepperidge Farm) Supreme	1/12 of 24-oz. cake	27.0
Pound (Sara Lee):		
Regular	1/10 of 10¾-oz. cake	14.2
Banana nut	1/10 of 11-oz.- cake	15.1
Chocolate	1/10 of 10¾-oz. cake	14.4
Homestyle	1/10 of 9½-oz. cake	13.1
Spice (Weight Watchers)	2⅝-oz. serving	27.2
Strawberry cream		
(Pepperidge Farm) Supreme	1/12 of 12-oz. cake	27.0
Strawberries 'n cream, layer		
(Sara Lee)	⅛ of 20½-oz. cake	29.4
Torte (Sara Lee):		
Apples'n cream	⅛ of 21-oz. cake	26.2
Fudge & nut	⅛ of 15¾-oz. cake	21.0
Vanilla (Pepperidge Farm) layer	1/10 of 17-oz. cake	25.0
Walnut, layer (Sara Lee)	⅛ of 18-oz. cake	22.8
CAKE OR COOKIE ICING		
(Pillsbury) all flavors	1 T.	12.0
CAKE ICING:		
Butter pecan (Betty Crocker)		
Creamy Deluxe	1/12 of can	27.0
Caramel pecan (Pillsbury)		
Frosting Supreme	1/12 of can	21.0
Cherry (Betty Crocker)		
Creamy Deluxe	1/12 of can	28.0
Chocolate:		
(Betty Crocker) *Creamy Deluxe:*		
Regular or sour cream	1/12 of can	25.0
Chip	1/12 of can	27.0
Milk	1/12 of can	26.0
(Duncan Hines)	1/12 of can	25.0
(Pillsbury) *Frosting Supreme:*		
Fudge	1/12 of can	24.0
Milk	1/12 of can	23.0
Coconut almond (Pillsbury) *Frosting*		
Supreme	1/12 of can	17.0
Cream cheese:		
(Betty Crocker) *Creamy Deluxe*	1/12 of can	27.0
(Pillsbury) *Frosting Supreme*	1/12 of can	27.0
Double dutch (Pillsbury) *Frosting*		
Supreme	1/12 of can	22.0
Lemon (Pillsbury)		
Frosting Supreme	1/12 of can	26.0
Orange (Betty Crocker)		
Creamy Deluxe	1/12 of can	28.0

Food and Description	*Measure or Quantity*	*Carbohydrates (grams)*
Strawberry (Pillsbury) *Frosting Supreme*	1/12 of can	26.0
Vanilla:		
(Betty Crocker) *Creamy Deluxe*	1/12 of can	28.0
(Duncan Hines)	1/12 of can	25.5
(Pillsbury) *Frosting Supreme*	1/12 of can	27.0
White:		
Home recipe, boiled	4 oz.	91.1
Home recipe, uncooked	4 oz.	92.5
(Betty Crocker) *Creamy Deluxe*, sour cream	1/12 of can	27.0
***CAKE ICING MIX:**		
Regular:		
Banana (Betty Crocker) *Chiquita*, creamy	1/12 of pkg.	30.0
Butter Brickle (Betty Crocker) creamy	1/12 of pkg.	30.0
Butter pecan (Betty Crocker) creamy	1/12 of pkg.	30.0
Caramel (Pillsbury) *Rich'n Easy*	1/12 of pkg.	24.0
Chocolate:		
Home recipe, fudge	1/2 cup	103.8
(Betty Crocker) creamy:		
Fluffy, almond fudge	1/12 of pkg.	27.0
Fudge, creamy, dark or milk	1/12 of pkg.	30.0
(Pillsbury) *Rich'n Easy*, fudge or milk	1/12 of pkg.	26.0
Coconut almond (Pillsbury)	1/12 of pkg.	16.0
Coconut pecan:		
(Betty Crocker) creamy	1/12 of pkg.	18.0
(Pillsbury)	1/12 of pkg.	20.0
Cream cheese & nut (Betty Crocker) creamy	1/12 of pkg.	24.0
Lemon:		
(Betty Crocker) *Sunkist*, creamy	1/12 of pkg.	30.0
(Pillsbury) *Rich'n Easy*	1/12 of pkg.	25.0
Strawberry (Pillsbury) *Rich'n Easy*	1/12 of pkg.	25.0
Vanilla, (Pillsbury) *Rich'n Easy*	1/12 of pkg.	25.0
White:		
(Betty Crocker) fluffy	1/12 of pkg.	16.0
(Betty Crocker) sour cream, creamy	1/12 of pkg.	31.0
(Pillsbury) fluffy	1/12 of pkg.	60.0
CAKE MIX:		
Regular:		
Angel food:		

Food and Description	*Measure or Quantity*	*Carbohydrates (grams)*
(Betty Crocker):		
Chocolate or one-step	1/12 pkg.	32.0
Traditional	1/12 pkg.	30.0
(Duncan Hines)	1/12 of pkg.	28.9
*(Pillsbury) raspberry or white	1/12 of cake	32.0
Applesauce raisin (Betty Crocker)		
Snackin' Cake	1/9 of pkg.	33.0
*Applesauce spice (Pillsbury)	1/12 of cake	33.0
Banana:		
*(Betty Crocker) *Supermoist*	1/12 of cake	36.0
*(Pillsbury) *Pillsbury Plus*	1/12 of cake	36.0
Banana walnut (Betty Crocker)		
Snackin' Cake	1/9 pkg.	31.0
*Boston cream (Pillsbury) *Bundt*	1/16 of cake	43.0
*Butter (Pillsbury):		
Pillsbury Plus	1/12 of cake	36.0
Streusel Swirl, rich	1/16 of cake	38.0
**Butter Brickle* (Betty Crocker)		
Supermoist	1/12 of cake	37.0
*Carrot (Betty Crocker)		
Supermoist	1/12 of cake	34.0
*Carrot'n spice (Pillsbury)		
Pillsbury Plus	1/12 of cake	36.0
*Cheesecake:		
(Jello-O)	1/8 of 8" cake	36.5
(Royal)	1/8 of cake	31.0
*Cherry chip (Betty Crocker)		
Supermoist	1/12 of cake	36.0
Chocolate:		
(Betty Crocker):		
*Pudding	1/6 of cake	45.0
Snackin' Cake:		
Almond	1/9 pkg.	31.0
Fudge Chip	1/9 pkg.	32.0
Stir 'N Frost:		
With chocolate frosting	1/6 pkg.	40.0
Fudge, with vanilla frosting	1/6 pkg.	41.0
Superpmoist:		
*Fudge	1/12 of cake	35.0
*Milk	1/12 of cake	36.0
*(Pillsbury):		
Bundt:		
Fudge nut crown	1/16 of cake	31.0
Fudge, tunnel	1/16 of cake	30.0
Macaroon	1/16 of cake	37.0

Food and Description	*Measure or Quantity*	*Carbohydrates (grams)*
Pillsbury Plus:		
Fudge, dark	1/12 of cake	35.0
Fudge, marble	1/12 of cake	36.0
Streusel Swirl, German	1/16 of cake	36.0
*Cinnamon (Pillsbury)		
Streusel Swirl	1/16 of cake	38.0
Coconut pecan (Betty Crocker)		
Snackin' Cake	1/9 of pkg.	30.0
Coffee cake:		
*(Aunt Jemima)	1/8 of cake	29.8
*(Pillsbury)		
Apple cinnamon	1/8 of cake	40.0
Cinnamon streusel	1/8 of cake	41.0
Date nut (Betty Crocker)		
Snackin' Cake	1/9 of pkg.	32.0
Devil's food:		
*(Betty Crocker) *Supermoist*	1/12 of cake	34.0
(Duncan Hines) deluxe	1/12 of pkg.	35.6
*(Pillsbury) *Pillsbury Plus*	1/12 of cake	35.0
Fudge (See Chocolate)		
Golden chocolate chip		
(Betty Crocker) *Snackin' Cake*	1/9 of pkg.	34.0
Lemon:		
(Betty Crocker):		
*Chiffon	1/12 of cake	35.0
Stir 'N Frost, with		
lemon frosting	1/12 of pkg.	45.0
Supermoist	1/12 of cake	36.0
*(Pillsbury):		
Bundt, tunnel of	1/16 of cake	45.0
Streusel Swirl	1/16 of cake	36.0
*Lemon blueberry (Pillsbury)		
Bundt	1/16 of cake	28.0
Marble:		
*(Betty Crocker) *Supermoist*	1/12 of cake	36.0
*(Pillsbury):		
Bundt, supreme, ring	1/16 of cake	38.0
Streusel Swirl, fudge	1/16 of cake	38.0
*Oats'n brown sugar (Pillsbury)		
Pillsbury Plus	1/12 of cake	35.0
*Orange (Betty Crocker)		
Supermoist	1/12 of cake	36.0
Pound:		
*(Betty Crocker) golden	1/12 of cake	27.0
*(Dromedary)	3/4" slice	29.0
*(Pillsbury) *Bundt*	1/16 of cake	33.0

Food and Description	*Measure or Quantity*	*Carbohydrates (grams)*
Spice (Betty Crocker):		
Snackin' Cake, raisin	1/9 pkg.	32.0
Stir 'N Frost, with vanilla frosting	1/6 of cake	47.0
Supermoist	1/12 of cake	36.0
Strawberry:		
*(Betty Crocker) *Supermoist*	1/12 of cake	36.0
*(Pillsbury) *Pillsbury Plus*	1/12 of cake	37.0
*Upside down (Betty Crocker) pineapple	1/9 of cake	43.0
White:		
*(Betty Crocker):		
Stir 'N Frost, with chocolate frosting	1/6 of cake	38.0
Supermoist	1/12 of cake	35.0
(Duncan Hines) deluxe	1/12 of pkg.	36.1
*(Pillsbury) *Pillsbury Plus*	1/12 of cake	35.0
Yellow:		
*(Betty Crocker) *Supermoist*	1/12 of cake	36.0
(Duncan Hines) deluxe	1/12 of pkg.	37.0
*(Pillsbury) *Pillsbury Plus*	1/12 of cake	36.0
*Dietetic:		
Chocolate (Dia-Mel; Estee)	1/10 of cake	17.0
Lemon (Dia-Mel)	1/10 of cake	18.0
White (Estee)	1/10 of cake	18.0
CAMPARI, 45 proof	1 fl. oz.	7.1
CANDY, REGULAR:		
Almond, chocolate covered (Hershey's) *Golden Almond*	1 oz.	12.4
Almond, Jordan (Banner)	1¼-oz. box	27.9
Baby Ruth	1.8-oz. piece	31.0
Bridge Mix (Nabisco)	1 piece	1.4
Butterfinger	1.6-oz. bar	28.0
Butterscotch Skimmers (Nabisco)	1 piece	5.7
Caramel:		
Caramel Flipper (Wayne)	1 oz.	19.0
Caramel Nip (Pearson)	1 piece	5.6
Charleston Chew	1½-oz. bar	32.6
Cherry, chocolate-covered (Nabisco; *Welch's*)	1 piece	13.0
Chocolate bar:		
Crunch (Nestlé)	1 1/16-oz. bar	19.1
Milk:		
(Hershey's)	1.2-oz. bar	19.4
(Hershey's)	4-oz. bar	64.7
(Nestlé)	.35-oz. bar	6.0

Food and Description	*Measure or Quantity*	*Carbohydrates (grams)*
(Nestlé)	1¹⁄₁₆-oz. bar	18.1
Special Dark (Hershey's)	1.05-oz. bar	18.4
Special Dark (Hershey's)	4-oz. bar	70.2
Chocolate bar with almonds:		
(Hershey's) milk	.35-oz. bar	5.4
(Hershey's) milk	1.15-oz. bar	17.6
(Nestlé)	1-oz.	17.0
Chocolate Parfait (Pearson)	1 piece	5.2
Chuckles	1 oz.	23.0
Clark Bar	1.4-oz. bar	28.4
Coffee Nip (Pearson)	1 piece	5.6
Coffioca (Pearson)	1 piece	5.2
Crispy Bar (Clark)	1¼-oz. bar	24.2
Crows (Mason)	1 piece	2.7
Dots (Mason)	1 piece	2.7
Dutch Treat Bar (Clark)	1⅙-oz. bar	20.3
Fudge (Nabisco) bar, *Home Style*	1 bar	13.9
Good & Plenty	1 oz	24.8
Halvah (Sahadi) original and marble	1 oz.	13.0
Jelly bean (Curtiss)	1 piece	3.0
Jelly rings, *Chuckles*	1 piece	9.0
Jujubes, Chuckles	1 piece	3.3
Ju Jus:		
Assorted	1 piece	2.0
Coins or raspberries	1 piece	4.0
Kisses (Hershey's)	1 piece (.2 oz.)	2.8
Kit Kat	.6-oz. bar	9.4
Krackel Bar	.35-oz. bar	5.9
Krackel Bar	1.2-oz. bar	20.3
Licorice:		
Licorice Nips (Pearson)	1 piece	5.6
(Switzer) bars, bites or stix:		
Black	1 oz.	22.1
Cherry or strawberry	1 oz.	23.2
Chocolate	1 oz.	22.7
Life Savers, drop	1 piece	2.3
Life Savers, mint	1 piece	1.7
Lollipops (Life Savers)	.9-oz. pop	24.0
Mallo Cup (Boyer)	9 16-oz. piece	11.2
Malted milk balls (Brach's)	1 piece	.9
Mars Bar (M&M/Mars)	1½-oz. serving	29.4
Marshmallow (Campfire)	1 oz.	24.9
Mary Jane (Miller):		
Small size	¼ oz.	3.5
Large size	1½-oz. bar	20.3
Milk Duds (Clark)	¾-oz. box	17.8

Food and Description	*Measure or Quantity*	*Carbohydrates (grams)*
Milky Way (M&M/Mars)	.8-oz. bar	42.2
Mint or peppermint:		
Jamaica or Liberty Mints (Nabisco)	1 piece	5.8
Mint Parfait (Pearson)	1 piece	5.2
Junior mint pattie (Nabisco)	1 piece	2.0
M&M's:		
Peanut	1.7-oz. pkg.	32.3
Plain	1.69-oz. pkg.	32.6
Mr. Goodbar (Hershey's)	.35-oz. bar	4.9
Mr. Goodbar (Hershey's)	1½-oz. bar	20.8
$100,000 Bar (Nestle)	1¼-oz. bar	23.8
Orange slices (Curtiss)	1 piece	1.0
Peanut, chocolate-covered (Nabisco)	1 piece	1.6
Peanut brittle (Planters):		
Jumbo Peanut Block Bar	1 oz.	23.0
Jumbo Peanut Block Bar	1 piece (4 grams)	12.0
Peanut butter cup:		
(Boyer)	1.5-oz. pkg.	17.4
(Reese's)	.6-oz. cup	8.7
Raisin, chocolate-covered (Nabisco)	1 piece	.6
Reggie Bar	2-oz. bar	29.0
Rolo (Hershey's)	1 piece	4.1
Royals, mint chocolate (M&M/Mars)	1½-oz. serving	21.2
Sesame Crunch (Sahadi)	¾-oz. bar	7.0
Snickers	1.8-oz. bar	33.5
Spearmint leaves:		
(Curtiss)	1 piece	8.0
(Nabisco) *Chuckles*	1 piece	6.6
Starburst (M&M/Mars)	1-oz. serving	24.2
Sugar Babies (Nabisco)	1 piece	1.3
Sugar Daddy (Nabisco):		
Caramel sucker	1 piece	26.4
Nugget	1 piece	6.0
Sugar Mama (Nabisco)	1 piece	18.6
Summit, cookie bar (M&M/Mars)	1 oz.	12.0
Taffy, turkish (Bonomo)	1 oz.	24.4
3 Musketeers	.8-oz. bar	17.3
3 Musketeers	2-oz. serving	44.6
Tootsie Roll:		
Chocolate	23-oz. midgee	5.3
Chocolate	1/16-oz. bar	14.3
Chocolate	1-oz. bar	22.9
Flavored	.6-oz. square	3.8
Pop, all flavors	.49-oz. pop	12.5

Food and Description	*Measure or Quantity*	*Carbohydrates (grams)*
Pop drop, all flavors	4.7-gram piece	4.2
Twix, cookie bar (M&M/Mars)	1¾-oz. serving	32.6
Twix, peanut butter cookie bar (M&M/Mars)	1¾-oz. serving	27.9
Twizzler:		
Cherry, chocolate or strawberry	1 oz.	22.0
Licorice	1 oz.	20.0
Whatchamacallit (Hershey's)	1.15-oz. bar	18.7
World Series Bar	1 oz.	21.3
Zagnut Bar (Clark)	.7-oz. bar	14.6
CANDY, DIETETIC:		
Carob bar, *Joan's Natural:*		
Coconut	3-oz. bar	28.4
Fruit & nut	3-oz. bar	31.2
Honey bran	3-oz. bar	34.0
Peanut	3-oz. bar	27.4
Chocolate or chocolate flvaored bar:		
Coconut (Estee)	.2-oz. square	2.0
Coffee (Louis Sherry)	.2-oz. square	2.0
Crunch (Estee)	.2-oz. square	2.0
Fruit & nut (Estee)	.2-oz. square	2.5
Milk (Estee)	.2-oz. square	2.5
Orange (Louis Sherry)	.2-oz. square	2.0
Toasted bran (Estee)	.2-oz. square	2.5
Estee-ets, with peanuts (Estee)	1 piece	.8
Gum drops (Estee) any flavor	1 piece	.7
Lollipop (Estee; Louis Sherry)	1 piece	5.0
Mint:		
(Estee) all flavors	1 piece	1.0
(Sunkist):		
Mini mint	1 piece	.2
Roll mint	1 piece	.9
Peanut butter cup (Estee)	1 cup	3.3
Raisins, chocolate-covered (Estee)	1 piece	.7
CANNELLONI, frozen:		
(Stouffer's) cheese, with tomato sauce	9⅛-oz. pkg.	18.0
(Weight Watchers) florentine, one-compartment	13-oz. meal	52.0
CANTALOUPE, cubed	½ cup	6.1
CAPERS (Crosse & Blackwell)	1 tsp.	1.0
CAP'N CRUNCH, cereal (Quaker):		
Regular or crunchberry	¾ cup	22.9
Peanut butter	¾ cup	20.9
CAPOCOLLO (Hormel)	1 oz.	0.
CARAWAY SEED (French's)	1 tsp.	.8

Food and Description	Measure or Quantity	Carbohydrates (grams)
CARNATION INSTANT BREAKFAST:		
Bar:		
Chocolate chip or chocolate crunch	1 bar	20.0
Honey nut	1 bar	18.0
Packets, all flavors	1 packet	23.0
CARROT:		
Raw	5½′ × 1″ piece	4.8
Boiled, slices	½ cup	5.4
Canned, regular pack solids & liq.:		
(Del Monte)	½ cup	7.0
(Libby's) diced	½ cup	4.1
(Stokely-Van Camp) diced	½ cup	6.0
Canned, dietetic pack, solids & liq.:		
(Featherweight)	½ cup	6.0
(S&W) *Nutradiet*, slices	½ cup	7.0
Frozen:		
(Birds Eye) whole, baby, deluxe	⅓ pkg.	9.1
(Green Giant) cuts, in butter sauce	½ cup	16.0
(McKenzie)	⅓ pkg.	9.0
CASABA MELON	1-lb. melon	14.7
CASHEW NUT:		
(Fisher) dry or oil roasted	1 oz.	8.2
(Planters):		
Dry roasted	1 oz.	9.0
Oil roasted	1 oz.	8.0
CATSUP:		
Regular:		
(Del Monte)	1 T.	3.9
(Smucker's)	1 T.	4.5
Dietetic or low calorie:		
(Del Monte) No Salt Added	1 T.	4.0
(Featherweight)	1 T.	1.0
(Tillie Lewis) *Tasti Diet*	1 T.	2.0
CAULIFLOWER:		
Raw or boiled buds	½ cup	2.6
Frozen:		
(Birds Eye):		
Regular	⅓ pkg.	4.6
With cheese sauce	⅓ pkg.	8.2
(Green Giant) in cheese sauce	½ cup	10.0
(Seabrook Farms)	⅓ pkg.	4.5
CAVIAR:		
Pressed	1 oz.	1.4

Food and Description	*Measure or Quantity*	*Carbohydrates (grams)*
Whole eggs	1 T.	.5
CELERY:		
1 large outer stalk	8″ × 1½″ at root end	1.6
Diced or cut	½ cup	2.1
Salt (French's)	1 tsp.	Tr.
Seed (French's)	1 tsp.	1.1
CERTS	1 piece	1.5
CERVELAT (Hormel) Viking	1 oz.	0.
CHABLIS WINE:		
(Great Western)	3 fl. oz.	2.3
(Louis M. Martini)	3 fl. oz.	.2
(Paul Masson) regular or light	3 fl. oz.	2.7
CHAMPAGNE:		
(Great Western):		
Regular	3 fl. oz.	2.4
Brut	3 fl. oz.	3.4
Pink	3 fl. oz.	4.9
(Taylor) dry	3 fl. oz.	3.9
CHARDONNAY WINE		
(Louis M. Martini)	3 fl. oz.	.2
CHARLOTTE RUSSE,		
home recipe	4 oz.	38.0
CHEERIOS, cereal, (General Mills):		
Regular	1¼ cups	20.0
Honey-nut	¾ cup	23.0
CHEESE:		
American or cheddar:		
Cube, natural	1″ cube	.4
(Featherweight) low sodium	1 oz.	1.0
Laughing Cow	1 oz.	Tr.
(Sargento)	1 oz.	1.0
Blue:		
(Frigo)	1 oz.	1.0
Laughing Cow:		
Cube	⅙ oz.	.1
Wedge	¾ oz.	.5
(Sargento) cold pack or crumbled	1 oz.	1.0
Bonbino, *Laughing Cow*	1 oz.	Tr.
Brick (Sargento)	1 oz.	1.0
Brie (Sargento) *Danish Danko*	1 oz.	.1
Burgercheese (Sargento)		
Danish Danko	1 oz.	1.0
Camembert (Sargento)		
Danish Danko	1 oz.	88
Colby:		
(Featherweight) low sodium	1 oz.	0.

Food and Description	*Measure or Quantity*	*Carbohydrates (grams)*
(Pauly) low sodium	1 oz.	.6
(Sargento) shredded or sliced	1 oz.	1.0
Cottage:		
Unflavored:		
(Bison) regular or dietetic	1 oz.	1.0
(Dairylea)	1 oz.	1.0
Flavored (Friendship):		
Dutch apple	1 oz.	2.5
Garden salad	1 oz.	1.0
Pineapple	1 oz.	3.8
Cream, plain, unwhipped (Friendship)	1 oz.	.8
Edam:		
(House of Gold; Sargento)	1 oz.	1.0
Laughing Cow	1 oz.	Tr.
Farmers (*Dutch Garden Brand*; Wispride)	1 oz.	1.0
Feta (Sargento) Danish, cups	1 oz.	1.0
Gjetost (Sargento) Norwegian	1 oz.	13.0
Gouda:		
(Frigo)	1 oz.	1.0
Laughing Cow	1 oz.	Tr.
Wispride	1 oz.	Tr.
Gruyere, *Swiss Knight*	1 oz.	Tr.
Havarti (Sargento) creamy or 60% mild	1 oz.	90
Hot pepper (Sargento)	1 oz.	1.0
Jarlsberg (Sargento) Norwegian	1 oz.	1.0
Kettle Moraine (Sargento)	1 oz.	1.0
Limburger (Sargento) natural	1 oz.	1.0
Monterey Jack (Frigo or Sargento)	1 oz.	1.0
Mozzarella:		
(Fisher) part skim milk	1 oz.	1.0
(Sargento):		
Bar, rounds, shredded regular or with spices, sliced for pizza or square	1 oz.	.3
Whole milk	1 oz.	1.0
Muenster:		
(Sargento) red rind	1 oz.	1.0
Wispride	1 oz.	Tr.
Parmesan:		
(Frigo):		
Grated	1 T.	Tr.
Whole	1 oz.	1.0

Food and Description	*Measure or Quantity*	*Carbohydrates (grams)*
(Sargento):		
Grated, non-dairy	1 T.	2.3
Wedge	1 oz.	1.0
Pizza (Sargento) shredded or sliced	1 oz.	1.0
Pot (Sargento) regular, French onion or garlic	1 oz.	1.0
Provolone:		
(Frigo)	1 oz.	1.0
Laughing Cow:		
Cube	⅙ oz.	.1
Wedge	¾ oz.	.5
(Sargento) sliced	1 oz.	1.0
Ricotta:		
(Frigo) part skim milk	1 oz.	.9
(Sargento) part skim or whole milk	1 oz.	1.0
Romano (Sargento) wedge	1 oz.	1.0
Roquefort, natural	1 oz.	.6
Samsoe (Sargento) Danish	1 oz.	.2
Stirred curd (Frigo)	1 oz.	.3
String (Sargento)	1 oz.	1.0
Swiss:		
Fisher; Frigo	1 oz.	0.
(Sargento) domestic or Finland, sliced		1.0
Taco (Sargento) shredded	1 oz.	1.0
Washed curd (Frigo)	1 oz.	1.0
CHEESE FONDUE, *Swiss Knight*	1 oz.	1.0
CHEESE FOOD:		
American or cheddar:		
(Fisher) substitute, *Ched-O-Mate* or *Sandwich-Mate*	1 oz.	1.0
(Weight Watchers) colored or white	1-oz. slice	1.0
Wispride:		
Regular or with blue cheese	1 oz.	2.0
Hickory smoked	1 oz.	3.0
& port wine	1 oz.	Tr.
Cheez-ola (Fisher)	1 oz.	1.0
Cracker snack (Sargento)	1 oz.	2.0
Mun-chee (Pauly)	1 oz.	2.0
Pimiento (Pauly)	.8-oz. slice	.8
Pizza-Mate (Fisher)	1 oz.	1.0
Swiss (Pauly)	.8-oz. slice	1.6
CHEESE PUFFS, frozen (Durkee)	1 piece	3.0

Food and Description	*Measure or Quantity*	*Carbohydrates (grams)*
CHEESE SPREAD:		
American or cheddar:		
(Fisher)	1 oz.	2.0
Laughing Cow	1 oz.	.7
(Nabisco) *Snack Mate*	1 tsp	.4
Blue, *Laughing Cow*	1 oz.	.7
Cheese'n Bacon (Nabisco) *Snack Mate*	1 tsp.	.4
Gruyere, *Laughing Cow, La Vache Qui Rit*	1 oz.	.7
Pimiento:		
(Nabisco) *Snack Mate*	1 tsp.	.3
(Price's)	1 oz.	2.0
Sharp (Pauly)	.8 oz.	.9
Swiss, process (Pauly)	.8 oz.	1.2
CHEESE STRAW, frozen (Durkee)	1 piece	1.0
CHENIN BLANC WINE (Louis M. Martini)	3 fl. oz.	.2
CHERRY, SWEET:		
Fresh, with stems	½ cup	10.2
Canned, regular pack		
(Stokely-Van Camp) pitted, solids & liq.	½ cup	11.0
Canned, dietetic, solids & liq.:		
(Diet Delight) with pits, water pack	½ cup	.2
(Featherweight) water pack:		
Dark	½ cup	13.0
Light	½ cup	11.0
CHERRY, CANDIED	1 oz.	24.6
CHERRY DRINK:		
Canned:		
(Hi-C)	6 fl. oz.	23.0
(Lincoln) cherry berry	6 fl. oz.	25.0
*Mix (Hi-C)	6 fl. oz.	18.0
CHERRY HEERING (Hiram Walker)	1 fl. oz.	10.0
CHERRY JELLY:		
Sweetened (Smucker's)	1 T.	13.5
Dietetic:		
(Featherweight)	1 T.	4.0
(Slenderella)	1 T.	6.0
CHERRY LIQUEUR (DeKuyper)	1 fl. oz.	8.5
CHERRY PRESERVE OR JAM:		
Sweetened (Smucker's)	1 T.	13.5
Dietetic (Dia-Mel)	1 T.	0.

Food and Description	*Measure or Quantity*	*Carbohydrates (grams)*
CHESTNUT, fresh, in shell	¼ lb.	38.6
CHEWING GUM:		
Sweetened:		
Beechies, Chiclets, tiny size	1 piece	1.6
Beech Nut; Beeman's, Big Red; Black Jack; Clove; Doublemint; Freedent; Fruit Punch; Juicy Fruit, Spearmint (Wrigley's); *Teaberry*	1 stick	2.3
Dentyne	1 piece	1.2
Hubba Bubba (Wrigley's)	1 piece	5.8
Dietetic:		
Bazooka, sugarless	1 piece	Tr.
(Clark; *Care*Free*)	1 piece	1.7
(Estee) bubble or regular	1 piece	1.4
(Featherweight) bubble or regular	1 piece	1.0
Orbit (Wrigley's)	1 piece	Tr.
CHEX, cereal (Ralston Purina):		
Rice	1 cup	25.0
Wheat	⅔ cup	23.0
Wheat & raisins	¾ cup	31.0
CHIANTI WINE (Italian Swiss Colony)	3 fl. oz.	1.5
CHICKEN:		
Broiler, cooked, meat only	3 oz.	0.
Fryer, fried, meat & skin	3 oz.	2.4
Fryer, fried, meat only	3 oz.	1.1
Fryer, fried, a 2½ lb. chicken (weighed with bone before cooking) will give you:		
Back	1 back	2.7
Breast	½ breast	1.2
Leg or drumstick	1 leg	.4
Neck	1 neck	2.0
Rib	1 rib	.8
Thigh	1 thigh	1.3
Wing	1 wing	.8
Fried skin	1 oz.	2.6
Hen & cock:		
Stewed, meat & skin	3 oz.	0.
Stewed, dark meat only	3 oz.	0.
Stewed, light meat only	3 oz.	0.
Stewed, diced	½ cup	0.
Roaster, roasted, dark or light meat, without skin	3 oz.	0.

Food and Description	Measure or Quantity	Carbohydrates (grams)
CHICKEN À LA KING:		
Home recipe	1 cup	12.3
Canned (Swanson)	½ of 10½-oz. can	9.0
Frozen:		
(Banquet) *Cookin' Bag*	5-oz. pkg.	10.0
(Green Giant) with biscuits	9-oz. entree	40.0
(Stouffer's) with rice	½ of 9½-oz. pkg.	38.0
(Weight Watchers)	9-oz. pkg.	7.0
CHICKEN BOUILLON:		
(Herb-Ox):		
Cube	1 cube	.6
Packet	1 packet	1.9
Low sodium (Featherweight)	1 tsp.	2.0
CHICKEN, BONED, CANNED	Any quantity	0.
CHICKEN CREAMED, frozen (Stouffer's)	6½ oz.	5.9
CHICKEN DINNER OR ENTREE:		
Canned (Swanson) & dumplings	7½ oz.	19.0
Frozen:		
(Banquet):		
American Favorites	11-oz. dinner	46.0
Extra Helping:		
& dressing	19-oz. dinner	89.0
Fried	17-oz. dinner	92.0
(Green Giant):		
Baked:		
In BBQ sauce with corn on cob	1 meal	45.0
Stir fry, & cashews	1 meal	37.0
Twin pouch, & broccoli with rice in cheese sauce	1 meal	26.0
(Morton):		
Regular:		
Boneless	10-oz. dinner	24.0
Sliced	5-oz. pkg.	7.0
Country Table, fried	15-oz. dinner	96.0
(Stouffer's):		
Cacciatore, with spaghetti	11¼-oz. meal	29.0
Divan	8½-oz. serving	14.0
Glazed, with vegetable rice, *Lean Cuisine*	8½-oz. meal	23.0
(Swanson):		
Regular, in white wine sauce	8¼-oz. entree	8.0
Hungry Man:		
Boneless	19-oz. dinner	65.0

Food and Description	Measure or Quantity	Carbohydrates (grams)
Fried:		
White portion	15¼-oz. dinner	90.0
White portion with whipped potato	11¾-oz. entree	49.0
TV Brand, fried, barbecue	11¼-oz. dinner	50.0
3-course, fried	15-oz. dinner	53.0
(Weight Watchers):		
Cacciatore	10-oz. serving	30.1
Oriental style	9½-oz. serving	27.5
Parmigiana, 2-compartment	7¾-oz. serving	11.0
Sliced in celery sauce, 2-compartment	8½-oz. serving	14.9
Southern fried patty, 2-compartment	6¾-oz. serving	11.0
CHICKEN FRICASEE	1 cup	7.7
CHICKEN, FRIED, frozen:		
(Banquet):		
Assorted	2-lb. pkg.	100.0
Thigh & drumsticks	25-oz. pkg.	80.0
(Morton) assorted	2-lb. pkg.	165.0
(Swanson):		
Assorted	3¼-oz. serving	11.0
Breast portions	3¼-oz. serving	15.0
Nibbles	3¼-oz. serving	16.0
Take-out style	3¼-oz. serving	10.0
CHICKEN GIBLETS,	2.1 oz.	2.8
CHICKEN LIVER PUFF, frozen (Durkee)	½-oz. piece	3.0
CHICKEN & NOODLES, frozen:		
(Banquet)	12-oz. dinner	50.7
(Green Giant) with vegetables	9-oz. pkg.	38.0
(Stouffer's):		
Escalloped	5¾-oz. serving	13.0
Paprikash	10½-oz. serving	32.0
CHICKEN NUGGETS, frozen (Banquet)	12-oz. pkg.	56.0
CHICKEN, PACKAGED (Louis Rich) breast, oven roasted	1-oz. slice	Tr.
CHICKEN PATTY, frozen (Banquet) breaded & fried	12-oz. pkg.	52.0
CHICKEN PIE, frozen:		
(Banquet) regular	8-oz. pie	45.0
(Morton)	8-oz. pie	33.0
(Stouffer's)	10.-oz. pie	40.0

Food and Description	*Measure or Quantity*	*Carbohydrates (grams)*
(Swanson):		
Regular	8-oz. pie	40.0
Hungry Man	1-lb. pie	65.0
CHICKEN PUFF, frozen (Durkee)	½-oz. piece	3.0
CHICKEN SALAD (Carnation)	¼ of 7½-oz. can	3.8
CHICKEN SOUP (see SOUP, Chicken)		
CHICKEN SPREAD:		
(Hormel)	1 oz.	0.
(Swanson)	1 oz.	2.0
(Underwood) chunky	½ of 4¾-oz. can	2.7
CHICKEN STEW, canned:		
Regular:		
(Libby's) with dumplings	8 oz.	20.2
(Swanson)	7⅝-oz.	16.0
Dietetic (Dia-Mel)	8-oz. can	19.0
CHICKEN STICKS, frozen (Banquet) breaded, fried	12-oz. pkg.	60.0
CHICKEN STOCK BASE (French's)	1 tsp.	1.0
CHICK-FIL-A:		
Sandwich	5.4-oz. serving	40.2
Soup, hearty, breast of chicken:		
Small	8½ oz.	11.1
Large	14.3 oz.	19.3
CHICK'N QUICK, frozen (Tyson):		
Breast fillet	3 oz.	12.0
Breast pattie	3 oz.	11.0
Chick'N Cheddar	3 oz.	12.0
Cordon bleu	5 oz.	16.0
Hoagies, Italian	3 oz.	12.0
Kiev	5 oz.	16.0
CHILI OR CHILI CON CARNE:		
Canned, regular pack:		
Beans only (Hormel)	5-oz. serving	19.0
With beans:		
(Hormel) hot	7½-oz. serving	24.0
(Libby's)	7½-oz. serving	25.0
(Swanson)	7¾-oz. serving	28.0
Without beans:		
(Hormel) regular	½ of 15-oz. can	12.0
(Libby's)	7½ oz. serving	11.0
Canned, dietetic pack (Dia-Mel) with beans	8-oz. serving	31.0
Frozen, with beans (Weight Watchers) one-compartment	10-oz. pkg.	26.0

Food and Description	*Measure or Quantity*	*Carbohydrates (grams)*
CHILI SAUCE:		
(Del Monte)	¼ cup (2 oz.)	17.0
(Ortega) green	1 oz.	1.1
(Featherweight) dietetic	1 T.	2.0
CHILI SEASONING MIX:		
*(Durkee)	1 cup	31.2
(French's) *Chili-O*	2-oz. pkg.	5.0
(McCormick)	1.2-oz. pkg.	36.1
CHIVES	1 T.	.2
CHOCO-DILE (Hostess)	2-oz. piece	35.0
CHOCOLATE, BAKING:		
(Baker's):		
Bitter or unsweetened	1 oz.	8.6
Semi-sweet, chips	½ cup	31.7
Sweetened, *German*	1 oz.	17.3
(Hershey's):		
Bitter or unsweetened	1 oz.	6.8
Sweetened:		
Dark chips, regular or mini	1 oz.	17.8
Milk, chips	1 oz.	18.2
Semi-sweet, chips	1 oz.	17.3
(Nestlé):		
Bitter or unsweetened, *Choco-bake*	1-oz. packet	8.0
Sweet or semi-sweet, morsels	1 oz.	17.0
CHOCOLATE ICE CREAM (See ICE CREAM, Chocolate)		
CHOCOLATE SYRUP (See SYRUP, Chocolate)		
CHOP SUEY, frozen:		
(Banquet) beef:		
Buffet Supper	2-lb. pkg.	39.1
Dinner	12-oz. dinner	38.8
(Stouffer's) beef with rice	12-oz. pkg.	37.7
***CHOP SUEY SEASONING MIX** (Durkee)	1¾ cups	21.0
CHOWDER (See SOUP, Chowder)		
CHOW MEIN:		
Canned:		
(Hormel) pork, *Short Orders*	7½-oz. can	13.0
(La Choy):		
Regular:		
Beef or meatless	¾ cup	5.0
Chicken	¾ cup	6.0
*Bi-Pack:		
Beef	¾ cup	6.0

Food and Description	*Measure or Quantity*	*Carbohydrates (grams)*
Pork, shrimp or vegetable	¾ cup	7.0
Frozen:		
(Banquet) chicken	12-oz. dinner	38.8
(Green Giant) chicken	9-oz. entree	29.0
(La Choy):		
Chicken	12-oz. dinner	44.06
Shrimp	12-oz. dinner	47.0
(Stouffer's) *Lean Cuisine*, chicken with rice	11¼-oz. pkg.	36.0
CHOW MEIN SEASONING MIX (Kikkoman)	1⅛-oz. pkg.	13.8
CINNAMON, GROUND (French's)	1 tsp.	1.4
CITRUS COOLER DRINK, canned (Hi-C)	6 fl. oz.	23.0
CLAM:		
Raw, all kinds, meat only	1 cup (8 oz.)	13.4
Raw, soft, meat & liq.	1 lb. (weighed in shell)	5.3
Canned, meat only	7½-oz. can	2.2
Frozen:		
(Howard Johnson's) fried	5-oz. pkg.	32.0
(Mrs. Paul's) fried, light	5-oz. pkg.	40.0
CLAM JUICE (Snow)	½ cup	1.2
CLARET WINE:		
(Gold Seal)	3 fl. oz.	.4
(Taylor) 12.5% alcohol	3 fl. oz.	2.4
CLORETS, gum or mint	1 piece	1.3
COBBLER, FROZEN (Weight Watchers)	4⅜-oz. serving	26.0
COCOA:		
Dry, unsweetened:		
(Hershey's)	1 T.	2.0
(Sultanta)	1 T.	3.5
Mix, regular:		
(Alba '66) instant, all flavors	1 envelope	11.0
(Carnation) all flavors	1-oz. pkg.	23.0
(Hershey's):		
Hot	1 oz.	21.0
Instant	3 T.	17.0
(Nestlé) *Rich'n Creamy*	1 oz.	22.0
**Swiss Miss*, regular or with mini marshmallows	6 fl. oz.	21.0
Mix, dietetic:		
(Carnation) *70 Calorie*	¾-oz. packet	15.0
*(Estee)	6 fl. oz.	9.0
(Ovaltine), hot, reduced calorie	.45-oz. pkg.	50.0

Food and Description	*Measure or Quantity*	*Carbohydrates (grams)*
COCOA KRISPIES, cereal (Kellogg's)	¾ cup	25.0
COCOA PUFFS cereal (General Mills)	1 oz.	25.0
COCONUT:		
Fresh, meat only	2" × 2" × ½" piece	4.2
Grated or shredded, firmly packed	½ cup	6.1
Dried:		
(Baker's):		
Angel Flake	⅓ cup	10.6
Cookie	⅓ cup	10.4
Premium shred	⅓ cup	12.4
(Durkee) shredded	¼ cup	2.0
COCO WHEATS, cereal	1 T.	9.3
COD	Any quantity	0.
COFFEE:		
Regular:		
**Max-Pax; Maxwell House Electra Perk; Yuban, Yuban Electra Matic*	6 fl. oz.	0.
**Mellow Roast*	6 fl. oz.	2.0
Decaffeinated:		
**Brim* or *Sanka*, regular or electric perk	6 fl. oz.	0.
**Brim*, freeze-dried; *Decafe; Nescafé*	6 fl. oz.	1.0
Instant:		
**Mellow Roast*	6 fl. oz.	2.0
**Sunrise*; *Yuban*	6 fl. oz.	1.0
*Mix (General Foods) *International Coffee:*		
Café Amaretto	6 fl. oz.	7.0
Café Irish Creme	6 fl. oz.	8.3
Café Vienna	6 fl. oz.	10.3
Irish Mocha Mint	6 fl. oz.	7.4
Suisse Mocha	6 fl. oz.	7.6
COFFEE CAKE (See CAKE, Coffee)		
COLA SOFT DRINK (see SOFT DRINK, Cola)		
COLD DUCK WINE		
(Great Western) pink	3 fl. oz.	7.7
COLESLAW, solids & liq., made with mayonnaise-type salad dressing	1 cup	8.3
***COLESLAW MIX** (Libby's)		
Super Slaw	½ cup	11.0

Food and Description	*Measure or Quantity*	*Carbohydrates (grams)*
COLLARDS:		
Leaves, cooked	⅓ pkg.	4.8
Canned (Sunshine) chopped, solids liq.	½ cup	3.8
Frozen, chopped:		
(Birds Eye)	⅓ pkg.	4.4
(McKenzie)	⅓ pkg.	4.0
(Southland)	⅓ of 16-oz. pkg.	5.0
COMPLETE CEREAL (Elam's)	1 oz.	17.5
CONCORD WINE:		
(Gold Seal)	3 fl. oz.	9.8
(Mogan David) dry	3 fl. oz.	1.8
COOKIE, REGULAR:		
Almond Windmill (Nabisco)	1 piece	7.0
Animal:		
(Dixie Belle)	1 piece	1.5
(Keebler):		
Regular	1 piece	1.9
Iced	1 piece	3.9
(Nabisco) *Barnum's Animals*	1 piece	1.9
Apple (Pepperidge Farm)	1 piece	7.6
Apple Crisp (Nabisco)	1 piece	7.0
Apple Spice (Pepperidge Farm)	1 piece	7.6
Apricot Raspberry (Pepperidge Farm)	1 piece	7.6
Assortment:		
(Nabisco) *Mayfair:*		
Crown creme sandwich	1 piece	8.0
Fancy shortbread biscuit	1 piece	3.3
Filigree creme sandwich	1 piece	8.5
Mayfair creme sandwich	1 piece	9.0
Tea rose creme	1 piece	7.7
(Pepperidge Farm):		
Butter	1 piece	7.0
Champagne	1 piece	4.0
Chocolate lace & Pirouette	1 piece	3.5
Marseilles	1 piece	6.0
Seville	1 piece	7.0
Southport	1 piece	9.0
Bordeaux (Pepperidge Farm)	1 piece	5.3
Brown edge wafer (Nabisco)	1 piece	4.2
Brownie:		
(Pepperidge Farm) chocolate nut	.4-oz. piece	6.3
(Sara Lee) frozen	⅛ of 13-oz. pkg.	26.1
Brussles (Pepperidge Farm)	1 piece	6.6
Brussles Mint (Pepperidge Farm)	1 piece	8.3

Food and Description	*Measure or Quantity*	*Carbohydrates (grams)*
Butter (Nabisco)	1 piece	3.5
Cappucino (Pepperidge Farm)	1 piece	6.0
Caramel peanut log (Nabisco)		
Heyday	1 piece	13.0
Chessman (Pepperidge Farm)	1 piece	6.0
Chocolate & chocolate-covered:		
(Keebler) fudge stripes	1 piece	7.0
(Nabisco):		
Famous wafer	1 piece	4.6
Pinwheel, cake	1 piece	21.0
Snap	1 piece	2.8
Chocolate chip:		
(Keebler) *Rich'N Chips*	1 piece	10.0
(Nabisco):		
Chips Ahoy!	1 piece	7.0
Chocolate	1 piece	7.3
Cookie Little	1 piece	1.0
(Pepperidge Farm):		
Regular size	1 piece	6.7
Large size	1 piece	18.0
Coconut:		
(Keebler) chocolate drop	1 piece	9.4
(Nabisco) bar, *Bakers Bonus*	1 piece	5.3
Coconut Granola		
(Pepperidge Farm)	1 piece	6.7
Creme Stick (Dutch Twin)		
chocolate coated	1 piece	5.0
Date Nut Granola		
(Pepperidge Farm)	1 piece	6.7
Fig bar:		
(Keebler)	1 piece	14.0
(Nabisco):		
Fig Newtons	1 piece	11.0
Fig Wheats	1 piece	11.5
Gingerman (Pepperidge Farm)	1 piece	5.0
Gingernsnaps (Nabisco) old fashioned	1 piece	30
Granola (Pepperidge Farm) large	1 piece	120
Ladyfinger	3¼" × 1⅜" × 1⅛"	7.1
Lido (Pepperidge Farm)	1 piece	10.5
Macaroon, coconut (Nabisco)	1 piece	11.5
Marshmallow:		
(Nabisco):		
Mallomars	1 piece	8.5
Puffs, cocoa covered	1 piece	14.0
Sandwich	1 piece	5.7
Twirls cakes	1 piece	20.0

Food and Description	*Measure or Quantity*	*Carbohydrates (grams)*
Milano (Pepperidge Farm)	1 piece	7.0
Mint Milano (Pepperidge Farm)	1 piece	8.3
Molasses (Nabisco) *Pantry*	1 piece	9.5
Molasses Crisp (Pepperidge Farm)	1 piece	4.0
Nilla wafer (Nabisco)	1 piece	3.0
Oatmeal:		
(Keebler) old fashioned	1 piece	12.0
(Nabisco):		
Bakers Bonus	1 piece	12.0
Cookie Little	1 piece	1.0
(Pepperidge Farm):		
Irish	1 piece	6.7
Large	1 piece	18.0
Orange Milano (Pepperidge Farm)	1 piece	8.3
Orleans (Pepperidge Farm)	1 piece	3.6
Peanut & peanut butter (Nabisco):		
Biscos	1 piece	5.7
Creme pattie	1 piece	4.3
Nutter Butter	1 piece	9.0
Peanut brittle (Nabisco)	1 piece	6.3
Pecan Sandies (Keebler)	1 piece	9.3
Raisin (Nabisco) fruit biscuit	1 piece	12.0
Raisin bar (Keebler) iced	1 piece	11.0
Raisin Bran (Pepperidge Farm)	1 piece	6.7
Sandwich:		
(Keebler):		
Chocolate fudge	1 piece	12.0
Eflwich	1 piece	8.1
Pitter Patter	1 piece	12.0
(Nabisco):		
Cameo, creme	1 piece	10.5
Mystic mint	1 piece	11.0
Oreo	1 piece	7.3
Oreo, double stuff	1 piece	9.0
Vanilla, *Cookie Break*	1 piece	7.3
Shortbread or shortcake:		
(Nabisco):		
Cookie Little	1 piece	1.1
Lorna Doone	1 piece	5.0
Pecan	1 piece	8.5
(Pepperide Farm)	1 piece	8.5
Social Tea, biscuit (Nabisco)	1 piece	3.5
Spiced wafers (Nabisco)	1 piece	6.0
Spiced Windmill (Keebler)	1 piece	9.2
St. Moritz (Pepperidge Farm)	1 piece	6.6

Food and Description	*Measure or Quantity*	*Carbohydrates (grams)*
Sugar cookie (Nabisco) rings, *Bakers Bonus*	1 piece	10.5
Sugar wafer:		
(Dutch Twin) any flavor	1 piece	4.7
(Keebler) *Krisp Kreem*	1 piece	4.2
(Nabisco) *Biscos*	1 piece	2.6
Sunflower Raisin (Pepperidge Farm)	1 piece	6.3
Tahiti (Pepperidge Farm)	1 piece	8.5
Vanilla wafer (Keebler)	1 piece	2.6
Waffle creme (Dutch Twin)	1 piece	5.7
Zanzibar (Pepperidge Farm)	1 piece	4.3
COOKIE, DIETETIC (Estee):		
Chocolate Chip	1 piece	3.0
Coconut	1 piece	2.7
Oatmeal raisin	1 piece	3.0
Sandwich duplex	1 piece	5.0
Wafer, chocolate covered	1 piece	14.0
COOKIE CRISP, cereal, any flavor	1 cup	25.0
***COOKIE DOUGH:**		
Refrigerated (Pillsbury):		
Brownie, fudge	1/24 of pkg.	22.0
Chocolate chip, double chocolate or sugar	1 cookie	7.7
Frozen (Rich's):		
Chocolate chip	1 cookie	20.3
Oatmeal	1 cookie	18.3
Ranger or sugar	1 cookie	17.0
***COOKIE MIX:**		
Regular:		
Brownie:		
(Betty Crocker):		
Fudge, regular size	1/16 of pan	22.0
Walnut, family size	1/24 of pan	19.0
(Pillsbury) fudge, regular size	2″ sq. (1/16 of pkg.)	23.0
Chocolate chip:		
(Betty Crocker) *Big Batch*	1 cookie	8.0
(Duncan Hines)	1/36 of pkg.	9.1
(Quaker)	1 cookie	8.5
Macaroon, coconut (Betty Crocker)	1/24 of pkg.	10.0
Oatmeal:		
(Betty Crocker) *Big Batch*	1 cookie	8.5
(Duncan Hines) raisin	1 cookie	9.1
(Nestle) raisin	1 cookie	9.0
(Quaker)	1 cookie	9.4
Peanut butter (Duncan Hines)	1/36 pkg.	7.5

Food and Description	Measure or Quantity	Carbohydrates (grams)
Sugar:		
(Betty Crocker) *Big Batch*	1 cookie	9.0
(Duncan Hines) golden	1 cookie	8.4
Dietetic (Estee) brownie	2″ × 2″ piece	8.0
COOKING SPRAY, *Mazola No Stick*	2-second spray	0.
CORN:		
Fresh, on the cob, boiled	5″ × 1¾″ ear	16.2
Canned, regular pack, solids & liq.:		
(Del Monte) regular or No Salt Added:		
Cream style, golden, wet pack	½ cup	18.0
Whole kernel, vacuum pack	½ cup	22.0
(Green Giant):		
Cream style	4¼ oz.	21.0
Whole kernel	4¼ oz.	18.0
Whole kernel, *Mexicorn*	3½ oz.	18.0
(LeSueur) whole kernel	¼ of 17-oz. can	18.0
(Libby's):		
Cream style	½ cup	21.2
Whole kernel	½ cup	18.8
Canned, dietetic pack, solids & liq.:		
(Diet Delight) whole kernel	½ cup	15.0
(Featherweight) whole kernel	½ cup	16.0
(S&W) *Nutradiet*, cream style	½ cup	21.0
Frozen:		
(Birds Eye):		
On the cob:		
Farmside	4.4-oz. ear	28.7
Little Ears	2.3-oz. ear	15.0
Whole kernel	⅓ of pkg.	19.4
Whole kernel in butter sauce	⅓ of pkg.	17.3
(Green Giant):		
On the cob	5½″ ear	30.0
On the cob, *Nibbler*	3″ ear	16.0
Whole kernel, *Harvest Fresh*	½ cup	22.0
Whole kernel, *Niblets*, golden, in butter sauce	⅓ of pkg.	18.0
(McKenzie) on the cob	5″ ear	29.0
CORNBREAD:		
Home recipe:		
Corn pone	4 oz.	41.1
Spoon bread	4 oz.	19.2
*Mix:		
(Aunt Jemima)	⅛ of pkg.	34.0
(Dromedary)	2″ × 2″ piece	19.0
(Pillsbury) *Ballard*	⅛ of recipe	25.0

Food and Description	*Measure or Quantity*	*Carbohydrates (grams)*
***CORN DOGS,** frozen:*		
(Hormel)	1 piece	21.0
(Oscar Mayer)	4-oz. piece	27.9
CORNED BEEF:		
Cooked, boneless, medium fat	4 oz.	0.
Canned, regular pack:		
Dinty Moore (Hormel)	3 oz.	0.
(Libby's)	⅓ of 7-oz. can	2.0
Canned, dietetic (Featherweight) loaf	2½ oz.	0.
Packaged:		
(Eckrich) sliced	1-oz. slice	1.0
(Oscar Mayer) jellied loaf	1-oz. slice	0.
CORNED BEEF HASH, canned:		
(Libby's)	⅓ of 24-oz. can	21.0
Mary Kitchen (Hormel)	7½-oz. serving	19.0
CORNED BEEF HASH DINNER, frozen (Banquet)	10-oz. dinner	42.6
CORNED BEEF SPREAD (Underwood)	1 oz.	Tr.
CORN FLAKE CRUMBS (Kellogg's)	¼ cup	25.0
CORN FLAKES, cereal:		
(Featherweight) low sodium	1¼ cups	25.0
(General Mills) *Country*	1 cup	25.0
(Kellogg's):		
Regular	1 cup	25.0
Honey & Nut	¾ cup	24.0
Sugar Frosted	¾ cup	26.0
(Ralston Purina) regular or sugar frosted	1 cup	25.0
CORN MEAL:		
Bolted (Aunt Jemima/Quaker)	3 T.	22.2
Mix:		
(Aunt Jemima)	1 cup	124.8
(Elam's)	1 cup	99.6
CORNNUTS	1 oz.	21.0
CORNSTARCH (Argo; Kingsford's; Duryea)	1 tsp.	2.8
CORN SYRUP (see SYRUP, Corn)		
COUGH DROP:		
(Beech-Nut)	1 drop	2.5
(Pine Bros.)	1 drop	1.9
COUNT CHOCULA, cereal (General Mills)	1 oz. (1 cup)	24.0
CRAB:		
Fresh, steamed:		

Food and Description	*Measure or Quantity*	*Carbohydrates (grams)*
Whole	½ lb.	.6
Meat only	4 oz.	.6
Canned, king crab (Icy Point; Pillar Rock)	3¼ oz.	2.3
Frozen (Wakefield's)	4 oz.	.7
CRAB APPLE, flesh only	¼ lb.	20.2
CRAB APPLE JELLY (Smucker's)	1 T.	13.5
CRAB, DEVILED, frozen (Mrs. Paul's) breaded & fried	½ of 6-oz. pkg.	20.0
CRAB IMPERIAL, home recipe	1 cup	8.6
CRACKER, PUFFS & CHIPS:		
Arrowroot biscuit (Nabisco)	1 piece	3.5
Bacon'n Dip (Nabisco)	1 piece	.9
Bacon-flavored thins (Nabisco)	1 piece	1.2
Bacon toast (Keebler)	1 piece	2.0
Biscos (Nabisco)	1 piece	2.6
Bran wafer (Featherweight)	1 piece	2.0
Bugles (General Mills)	1 oz.	18.0
Cheese flavored:		
Cheddar triangles (Nabisco)	1 piece	.9
Cheese'n Crunch (Nabisco)	1 oz.	14.0
Chee-Tos, crunchy or puffed	1 oz.	15.0
Cheeze Balls (Planters)	1 oz.	15.0
Cheeze Curls (Planters)	1 oz.	15.0
Country Cheddar'n sesame (Nabisco)	1 piece	1.0
(Dixie Belle)	1 piece	.7
Nachips, Old El Paso	1 oz.	15.3
Nips (Nabisco)	1 piece	.7
(Ralston)	1 piece	.7
Swiss cheese (Nabisco)	1 piece	1.1
Tid-Bit (Nabisco)	1 oz.	.5
Twists (Bachman) baked	1 oz.	17.0
Chicken in a Biskit (Nabisco)	1 piece	1.1
Chip O'Cheddar, Flavor Kist, (Schulze and Burch)	1 oz.	17.0
Chippers (Nabisco)	1 piece	1.7
Chipsters (Nabisco)	1 piece	.3
Club cracker (Keebler)	1 piece	2.1
Corn chips:		
(Bachman) regular or BBQ	1 oz.	15.0
(Featherweight) low sodium	1 oz.	15.0
Fritos, regular or barbecue flavor	1 oz.	16.0
Corn & Sesame Chips (Nabisco)	1 piece	.9
Creme Wafer Stick (Nabisco)	1 piece	6.3

Food and Description	*Measure or Quantity*	*Carbohydrates (grams)*
Crown Pilot (Nabisco)	1 piece	13.0
Diggers (Nabisco)	1 piece	.5
English Water Biscuit (Pepperidge Farm)	1 piece	3.1
Escort (Nabisco)	1 piece	2.6
Goldfish (Pepperidge Farm):		
Thins	1 piece	1.1
Tiny	1 piece	.4
Graham:		
(Dixie Belle) sugar-honey coated	1 piece	2.6
Flavor Kist (Schulze and Burch) sugar-honey coated	1 piece	10.0
Honey Maid (Nabisco)	1 piece	5.5
Graham, chocolate or cocoa-covered:		
Fancy Dip (Nabisco)	1 piece	8.0
(Keebler)	1 piece	5.6
(Nabisco)	1 piece	7.0
Melba Toast (See MELBA TOAST)		
Milk Lunch Biscuit (Keebler)	1 piece	4.5
Mucho Macho Nacho, Flavor Kist (Schulze and Burch)	1 oz.	18.0
Oyster:		
(Dixie Belle)	1 piece	.6
(Keebler) *Zesta*	1 piece	.3
(Nabisco) *Dandy or Oysterettes*	1 piece	.5
Pumpernickel Toast (Keebler)	1 piece	2.1
Ritz (Nabisco)	1 piece	2.0
Roman Meal Wafer, boxed	1 piece	1.3
Royal Lunch (Nabisco)	1 piece	8.0
Rusk, *Holland* (Nabisco)	1 piece	7.5
Ry-Krisp:		
Natural or sesame	1 triple cracker	5.0
Seasoned	1 triple cracker	4.5
Saltine:		
(Dixie Belle) regular or unsalted	1 piece	2.0
Premium (Nabisco)	1 piece	2.0
Zesta (Keebler)	1 piece	2.0
Sesame:		
Butter flavored (Nabisco)	1 piece	1.9
(Pepperidge Farm)	1 piece	3.0
Sesame Wheats! (Nabisco)	1 piece	1.8
Shindigs (Keebler)	1 piece	.9
Snackers (Ralston)	1 piece	2.2
Snackin' Crisp (Durkee) *O & C*	1 oz.	15.0
Snacks Sticks (Pepperidge Farm):		
Cheese or sesame	1 piece	2.3

Food and Description	*Measure or Quantity*	*Carbohydrates (grams)*
Lightly salted, pumpernickel, or rye	1 piece	2.5
Sociables (Nabisco)	1 piece	1.3
Water Cracker (Carr's) small	1 piece	2.5
Tortilla chips:		
(Bachman) nacho, taco flavor or toasted	1 oz.	17.0
Buenos (Nabisco) nacho	1 piece	1.2
Doritos, nacho or taco	1 oz.	18.0
(Nabisco) regular and nacho	1 piece	1.3
(Nalley's)	1 oz.	14.0
Tostitos	1 oz.	17.0
Town House Cracker (Keebler)	1 piece	1.8
Triscuit (Nabisco)	1 piece	3.0
Twigs (Nabisco)	1 piece	1.6
Uneeda Biscuit (Nabisco) unsalted	1 piece	3.7
Unsalted (Estee)	1 piece	2.5
Waldorf (Keebler) low sodium	1 piece	2.3
Waverly Wafer (Nabisco)	1 piece	2.6
Wheat (Pepperidge Farm) cracked or hearty	1 piece	3.6
Wheat Chips (Nabisco)	1 piece	.5
Wheat Crisps (Keebler)	1 piece	1.7
Wheatmeal Biscuit (Carr's) small	1 piece	5.9
Wheat Snack (Dixie Belle)	1 piece	1.2
Wheat Snack, *Flavor Kist* (Schulze and Burch):		
Regular	1 oz.	16.0
Rye	1 oz.	17.0
Wild onion	1 oz.	18.0
Wheatsworth (Nabisco)	1 piece	1.8
Wheat Thins (Nabisco)	1 piece	1.2
Wheat Toast (Keebler)	1 piece	2.0
Wheat wafer (Estee) *6 Calorie*	1 piece	1.0
Wheat wafer (Featherweight) unsalted	1 piece	2.3
CRACKER CRUMBS, graham (Nabsico)	⅛ of 9″ pie shell	12.0
CRACKER MEAL (Nabisco)	½ cup	47.5
CRANAPPLE JUICE (Ocean Spray,) canned:		
Regular	6 fl. oz.	32.1
Dietetic	6 fl. oz.	7.4
CRANBERRY, fresh (Ocean Spray)	½ cup	6.1
CRANBERRY JUICE COCKTAIL:		
Canned (Ocean Spray):		

Food and Description	*Measure or Quantity*	*Carbohydrates (grams)*
Regular	6 fl. oz.	26.4
Dietetic	6 fl. oz.	8.3
*Frozen (Welch's)	6 fl. oz.	26.0
CRANBERRY-ORANGE RELISH (Ocean Spray)	2 oz.	25.8
CRANBERRY-RASPBERRY SAUCE (Ocean Spray) jellied	2 oz.	20.8
CRANBERRY SAUCE:		
Home recipe	4 oz.	52.0
Canned (Ocean Spray):		
Jellied	2 oz.	21.7
Whole berry	2 oz.	22.0
CRANGRAPE (Ocean Spray)	6 fl. oz.	26.3
CRAN-RASPBERRY SAUCE (Ocean Spray) jellied	2 oz.	20.8
CRANTASTIC JUICE DRINK (Ocean Spray)	6 fl. oz.	27.0
***CRAZY COW*, cereal** (General Mills)	1 cup	25.0
CREAM:		
Half & Half (Dairylea)	1 fl. oz.	1.0
Light, table or coffee (Sealtest) 16% fat	1 T.	.6
Light, whipping, 30% fat (Sealtest)	1 T.	45
Heavy whipping (Dairylea)	1 fl. oz.	1.0
Sour (Dairylea)	1 fl. oz.	1.0
Sour, imitation (Pet)	1 T.	1.0
Substitute (See CREAM SUBSTITUTE)		
CREAM PUFFS:		
Home recipe, custard filling	3½″ × 2″ piece	26.7
Frozen (Rich's) chocolate	1⅓-oz. piece	16.9
CREAMSICLE (Popsicle Industries)	2½-fl.-oz. piece	13.0
CREAM SUBSTITUTE:		
Coffee Mate (Carnation)	1 tsp.	1.1
Coffee Rich	½ oz.	2.1
Dairy Light (Alba)	2.8-oz. envelope	1.0
N-Rich	1½ tsp.	1.6
(Pet)	1 tsp.	1.0
CREAM, OF WHEAT cereal:		
*Instant	1 T.	8.8
Mix'n Eat, dry:		
Regular	1 packet	24.0
Baked apple & cinnamon, banana & spice or maple & brown sugar	1 packet	32.0
Quick	1 T.	8.8
Regular	2½ T.	8.8

Food and Description	*Measure or Quantity*	*Carbohydrates (grams)*
CREME DE BANANA LIQUEUR (Mr. Boston)	1 fl. oz.	12.0
CREME DE CACAO:		
(Hiram Walker)	1 fl. oz.	15.0
(Mr. Boston):		
Brown	1 fl. oz.	14.3
White	1 fl. oz.	12.0
CREME DE CASSIS (Mr. Boston)	1 fl. oz.	14.1
CREME DE MENTHE:		
(Bols)	1 fl. oz.	11.3
(Mr. Boston):		
Green	1 fl. oz.	16.0
White	1 fl. oz.	13.0
CREME DE NOYAUX (Mr. Boston)	1 fl. oz.	13.5
CREPE, frozen:		
(Mrs. Paul's):		
Crab	5½-oz. pkg.	24.6
Shrimp	5½-oz. pkg.	23.8
(Stouffer's):		
Chicken with mushroom sauce	8¼-oz. pkg.	19.0
Ham & asparagus	6¼-oz. pkg.	21.0
Spinach with cheddar cheese sauce	9½-oz. pkg.	30.0
CRISP RICE CEREAL:		
(Featherweight) low sodium	1 cup	26.0
(Ralston Purina)	1 cup	25.0
CRISPY WHEATS'N RAISINS, cereal (General Mills)	¾ cup	23.0
CROUTON:		
(Arnold):		
Bavarian or English style	½ oz.	9.5
French, Italian or Mexican style	½ oz.	9.2
(Kellogg's) *Croutettes*	⅔ cup	14.0
(Pepperidge Farm):		
Cheddar & romano or onion & garlic	.5 oz.	10.0
Cheese & garlic or seasoned	.5 oz.	9.0
C-3PO'S, cereal (Kellogg's)	¾ cup	24.0
CUCUMBER:		
Eaten with skin	8-oz. cucumber	7.4
Pared, 10-oz. cucumber	7½″ × 2″ pared	6.6
Pared	3 slices	.8
CUMIN SEED (French's)	1 tsp.	.7
CUPCAKE:		
Regular (Hostess):		
Chocolate	1 cupcake	29.8

Food and Description	*Measure or Quantity*	*Carbohydrates (grams)*
Orange	1 cupcake	26.8
Frozen (Sara Lee) yellow	1 cupcake	31.5
***CUPCAKE MIX** (Flako)	1 cupcake	25.0
CUP O' NOODLES (Nissin Foods):		
Beef	2½-oz. serving	39.2
Beef, twin pack	1.2-oz. serving	18.2
Beef onion	2½-oz. serving	36.8
Beef onion, twin pack	1.2-oz. serving	19.4
Chicken, twin pack	1.2-oz. serving	18.6
Shrimp	2½-oz. serving	40.0
CURACAO:		
(Bols)	1 fl. oz.	10.3
(Hiram Walker)	1 fl. oz.	11.8
CURRANT, DRIED (Del Monte) Zante	½ cup	53.0
CURRANT JELLY (Smucker's)	1 T.	13.5
CUSTARD:		
Chilled, *Swiss Miss*, chocolate or egg flavor	4-oz. container	23.0
*Mix, dietetic (Featherweight)	½ cup	15.0
C.W. POST, cereal, plain or with raisins	¼ cup	20.3

D

Food and Description	Measure or Quantity	Carbohydrates (grams)
DAIRY QUEEN/BRAZIER:		
Banana split	13.-5-oz. serving	103.0
Brownie Delight, hot fudge	9.4-oz. serving	85.0
Buster Bar	5¼-oz. piece	41.0
Chicken sandwich	7.8-oz. sandwich	46.0
Cone:		
Plain, any flavor:		
Small	3-oz. cone	22.0
Regular	5-oz. cone	38.0
Large	7½-oz. cone	57.0
Dipped, chocolate:		
Small	3¼-oz. cone	25.0
Regular	5½-oz. cone	42.0
Large	8¼-oz. cone	64.0
Dilly Bar	3-oz. piece	21.0
Double Delight	9-oz. serving	69.0
DQ Sandwich	2.1-oz. sandwich	24.0
Fish sandwich:		
Plain	6-oz. sandwich	41.0
With cheese	6¼-oz. sandwich	39.0
Float	14-oz. serving	82.0
Freeze, vanilla	12-oz. serving	89.0
French fries:		
Regular	2½-oz. serving	25.0
Large	4-oz. serving	40.0
Frozen desert	4-oz. serving	27.0
Hamburger:		
Plain	1 burger	33.0
With cheese, single	1 burger	34.0
Hot dog:		
Regular:		
Plain or with cheese	1 serving	21.0
With chili	4½-oz. serving	23.0

Food and Description	*Measure or Quantity*	*Carbohydrates (grams)*
Super:		
Plain	6.2-oz. serving	44.0
With cheese	6.9-oz. serving	45.0
With chili	7.7-oz. serving	47.0
Lettuce	½ oz.	Tr.
Malt, chocolate:		
Small	10¼-oz. serving	91.0
Regular	14¾-oz. serving	134.0
Large	20¾-oz. serving	187.0
Mr. Misty:		
Plain:		
Small	8¼-oz. serving	48.0
Regular	11.64-oz. serving	63.0
Large	15½-oz. serving	84.0
Kiss	3.14-oz. serving	17.0
Float	14.5-oz. serving	74.0
Freeze	14.5-oz. serving	94.0
Onion rings	3-oz. serving	31.0
Parfait	10-oz. serving	76.0
Peanut Butter Parfait	10¾-oz. serving	94.0
Shake, chocolate:		
Small	10¼-oz. serving	82.0
Regular	14¾-oz. serving	120.0
Large	20¾-oz. serving	168.0
Strawberry shortcake	11-oz. serving	100.0
Sundae, chocolate:		
Small	3¾-oz. serving	33.0
Regular	6¼-oz. serving	56.0
Large	8¾-oz. serving	78.0
DAIQUIRI COCKTAIL (Mr. Boson):		
Regular	3 fl. oz.	9.0
Strawberry	3 fl. oz.	12.0
DATE (Dromedary):		
Chopped	¼ cup	31.0
Pitted	5 dates	23.0
DE CHAUNAC WINE (Great Western) 12% alcohol	3 fl. oz.	2.4
DELI'S, frozen (Pepperidge Farm):		
Beef with barbecue sauce	4-oz. piece	30.0
Mexican style	4-oz. piece	27.0
Reubein in rye pastry	4-oz. piece	25.0
Savory chicken salad	4-oz. piece	26.0
Turkey, ham & cheese	4-oz. piece	24.0
DESSERT CUPS (Hostess)	¾-oz. piece	14.0
DILL SEED (French's)	1 tsp.	1.2

Food and Description	*Measure or Quantity*	*Carbohydrates (grams)*
DING DONG (Hostess)	1 cake	21.0
DINNER, FROZEN (See individual listings such as BEEF, CHICKEN, TURKEY, etc.)		
DIP:		
Avocado (Nalley's)	1 oz.	.9
Barbecue (Nalley's)	1 oz.	1.1
Blue cheese:		
(Dean) tang	1 oz.	2.3
(Nalley's)	1 oz.	.9
Clam (Nalley's)	1 oz.	1.1
Enchilada, *Fritos*	1 oz.	3.9
Guacamole (Nalley's)	1 oz.	.9
Jalapeno:		
Fritos	1 oz.	3.7
(Hain) natural	1 oz.	2.5
Onion (Dean) French	1 oz.	1.9
Onion bean (Hain) natural	1 oz.	3.6
DISTILLED LIQUOR, any brand any proof	1 fl. oz.	Tr.
DONUTZ, cereal (General Mills) chocolate	1 cup	23.0
DOUGHNUT (See also *WINCHELL'S*):		
Regular (Hostess):		
Chocolate coated	1-oz. piece	13.6
Cinnamon	1-oz. piece	14.5
Donettes, frosted	1 piece	6.0
Old fashioned, plain	1.5-oz. piece	23.0
Powdered	1-oz. piece	15.1
Frozen (Morton):		
Regular:		
Boston creme	2.3-oz. piece	28.0
Chocolate iced	1.5-oz. piece	20.0
Jelly	1.8-oz. piece	23.0
Donut Holes, vanilla	⅕ of 7¾-oz. pkg.	22.0
Morning Light, jelly	2.6-oz. serving	33.0
DRAMBUIE (Hiram Walker)	1 fl. oz.	11.0
DRUMSTICK, frozen:		
Ice Cream, in a cone:		
Topped with peanuts	1 piece	22.7
Topped with peanuts & cone bisque	1 piece	23.6
Ice Milk, in a cone:		
Topped with peanuts	1 piece	24.3

Food and Description	*Measure or Quantity*	*Carbohydrates (grams)*
Topped with peanuts & cone bisque	1 piece	25.2
DUMPLINGS, STUFFED, canned, dietetic:		
(Dia-Mel)	8-oz. serving	15.0
(Featherweight)	7½-oz. serving	18.0

E

Food and Description	*Measure or Quantity*	*Carbohydrates (grams)*
ECLAIR:		
Home recipe, with custard filling and chocolate icing	4-oz. piece	26.3
Frozen (Rich's) chocolate	1 piece	30.0
EEL, smoked, meat only	4 oz.	0.
EGG, CHICKEN:		
Raw:		
White only	1 large egg	.3
Yolk only	1 large egg	.1
Boiled	1 large egg	.4
Fried in butter	1 large egg	.1
Omelet, mixed with milk & cooked in fat	1 large egg	1.5
Poached	1 large egg	.4
Scrambled, mixed with milk & cooked in fat	1 large egg	1.5
EGG MIX (Durkee):		
Omelet:		
*With bacon	½ of pkg.	10.0
*Puffy	½ of pkg.	10.5
Scrambled:		
Plain	.8-oz. pkg.	4.0
With bacon	1.3-oz. pkg.	6.0
EGG NOG, dairy (Meadow Gold) 6% fat	½ cup	25.5
EGG NOG COCKTAIL (Mr. Boston) 15% alcohol	3 fl. oz.	18.9
EGGPLANT:		
Boiled	4 oz.	4.6
Frozen (Mrs. Paul's):		
Parmesan	5½-oz. serving	20.0
Sticks, breaded & fried	3½-oz. serving	27.3
EGG ROLL, frozen:		
(La Choy):		

Food and Description	*Measure or Quantity*	*Carbohydrates (grams)*
Chicken, meat or shrimp	.4-oz. roll	4.0
Lobster	.4-oz. roll	4.3
Meat & shrimp	.25-oz. roll	2.5
Shrimp	3-oz. roll	24.0
(Van de Kamp's) cantonese	10½-oz. meal	64.0
EGG, SCRAMBLED, FROZEN		
(Swanson) and sausage, with hashed brown potatoes, *TV Brand*	6½-oz. entree	17.0
EGG SUBSTITUTE:		
Egg Magic (Featherweight)	½ of envelope	1.0
**Scramblers* (Morningstar Farms)	1 egg substitute	1.5
Second Nature (Avoset)	3 T.	2.0
ENCHILADA, frozen:		
Beef:		
(Banquet):		
Buffet Supper	2-lb. pkg.	148.0
Dinner	12-oz. dinner	72.0
(Green Giant) Sonora style	12-oz. entree	48.0
(Hormel)	1 piece	17.0
(Swanson) *TV Brand*	15-oz. dinner	72.0
(Van de Kamp's):		
Dinner	12-oz. dinner	45.0
Entree, shredded	5½-oz. serving	16.0
Cheese:		
(Banquet) Extra Helping	21¼-oz. dinner	105.0
(Hormel)	1 piece	18.0
(Van de Kamp's)	12-oz. dinner	44.0
Chicken (Van de Kamp's)	7½-oz. pkg.	24.0
ENCHILADA SAUCE:		
Canned (Del Monte) hot or mild	½ cup	11.0
*Mix (Durkee)	½ cup	6.2
ENDIVE, CURLY OR ESCAROLE, cut	½ cup	1.4
ESPRESSO COFFEE LIQUEUR	1 fl. oz.	15.0

F

Food and Description	Measure or Quantity	Carbohydrates (grams)
FARINA:		
(Hi-O) dry, regular	¼ cup	33.6
Malt-O-Meal dry:		
Regular	1 oz.	21.0
Quick cooking	1 oz.	22.0
*(Pillsbury) made with water and salt	⅔ cup	17.0
FAT, COOKING	Any quantity	0.
FENNEL SEED (French's)	1 tsp.	1.3
FETTUCINI ALFREDO, frozen (Stouffer's)	5-oz. serving	19.0
FIG:		
Small	1½" fig	7.7
Canned, regular pack (Del Monte) whole, solids & liq.	½ cup	28.0
Canned, dietetic (Featherweight) Kadota, water pack	½ cup	15.0
Dried (Sun-Maid) Mission, regular or figlets	3-oz. serving	50.0
FIG JUICE (Sunsweet)	6 fl. oz.	30.0
FIGURINES (Pillsbury):		
All flavors but chocolate peanut butter	1 bar	10.5
Chocolate peanut butter	1 bar	9.0
FILBERT:		
Shelled	1 oz.	4.7
(Fisher) oil dipped, salted	½ cup	5.4
FISH CAKE, frozen (Mrs. Paul's):		
Breaded & fried	2-oz. piece	12.0
Thins, breaded & fried	½ of 10-oz. pkg.	25.0
FISH & CHIPS, frozen:		
(Banquet) *Man-Pleaser*	14-oz. dinner	97.0
(Swanson):		
Hungry Man	15¾-oz. dinner	87.0

Food and Description	*Measure or Quantity*	*Carbohydrates (grams)*
TV Brand	5-oz. entree	30.0
(Van de Kamp's) batter dipped, french fried	½ of 14-oz. pkg.	39.4
FISH DINNER, frozen:		
(Banquet)	8¾-oz. dinner	45.0
(Morton)	9-oz. dinner	22.0
(Mrs. Paul's) parmesan	½ of 10-oz. pkg.	16.0
(Stouffer's) *Lean Cuisine,* florentine	9-oz. pkg.	13.0
(Van de Kamp's) batter dipped, french fried	11-oz. dinner	39.0
(Weight Watchers) au gratin	9-oz. meal	14.0
FISH FILLET, frozen:		
(Mrs. Paul's):		
Batter fried, crunchy	2¼-oz. piece	13.5
Breaded & fried	2-oz. piece	11.0
(Van de Kamp's):		
Batter dipped, french fried	3-oz. piece	12.5
Country seasoned	2.4-oz. piece	10.5
Today's Catch	4-oz. serving	0.
FISH KABOBS, frozen:		
(Mrs. Paul's) light batter	⅓ pkg.	17.7
(Van de Kamp's) batter dipped, french fried	.4-oz. piece	1.6
FISH SEASONING (Featherweight)	¼ tsp.	Tr.
FISH STICK, frozen:		
(Mrs. Paul's):		
Batter fried	1 piece	5.3
Breaded & fried	1 piece	4.2
(Van de Kamp's) batter dipped, french fried	1-oz. piece	5.2
FIT'N FROSTY (Alba '77):		
Chocolate or marshmallow flavor	1 envelope	11.5
Strawberry	1 envelope	12.0
Vanilla	1 envelope	11.3
****FIVE ALIVE*** (Snow Crop)	6 fl. oz.	20.8
FLOUNDER:		
Baked	4 oz.	0.
Frozen:		
(Mrs. Paul's) fillets, breaded & fried	3-oz. piece	9.5
(Van de Kamp's) *Today's Catch*	4-oz. serving	0.
FLOUR:		
(Aunt Jemima) self-rising	¼ cup	23.6
Ballard, self-rising	¼ cup	21.8
Bisquick (Betty Crocker)	¼ cup	19.0

Food and Description	*Measure or Quantity*	*Carbohydrates (grams)*
Buckwheat, dark	¼ cup	17.6
(Elam's):		
Brown rice, whole grain	¼ cup	25.8
Buckwheat, pure	¼ cup	27.2
Pastry, whole wheat	¼ cup	24.9
Rye, whole grain	¼ cup	24.2
Soy, roasted	¼ cup	9.8
Gold Medal (Betty Crocker) all-purpose	¼ cup	21.8
La Pina	¼ cup	21.8
Pillsbury's Best:		
All-purpose	¼ cup	21.5
Sauce & gravy	2 T.	11.0
Self-rising	¼ cup	21.0
Presto, self-rising	¼ cup	21.6
Wondra	¼ cup	21.8
FOLLE BLANC WINE		
(Louis M. Martini) 12½% alcohol	3 fl. oz.	.2
FRANKEN*BERRY, cereal (General Mills)	1 cup	24.0
FRANKFURTER:		
(Eckrich):		
Beef, or meat	1.6-oz. frankfurter	3.0
Beef or meat, jumbo	2-oz. frankfurter	3.0
Cheese	2-oz. frankfurter	3.0
Meat	1.2-oz. frankfurter	2.0
(Hormel):		
Beef or meat	1.6-oz. frankfurter	1.0
Range Brand, Wrangler, smoked, beef	1 frankfurter	2.0
(Hygrade) beef, *Ball Park*	2-oz. frankfurter	Tr.
(Louis Rich) turkey	1.5-oz. frankfurter	1.0
(Oscar Mayer):		
Beef	1.6-oz. frankfurter	.9
Little Wiener	2" frankfurter	.2
Wiener	1.6-oz. frankfurter	.8
Wiener, with cheese	1.6-oz. frankfurter	.7
FRANKS-N-BLANKETS, frozen (Durkee)	1 piece	1.0
FRENCH TOAST, frozen:		
(Aunt Jemima) regular or cinnamon swirl	1 slice	13.6
(Swanson) with sausage, *TV Brand*	4½-oz. pkg.	28.0
FRITTERS, FROZEN (Mrs. Paul's):		
Apple	2-oz. piece	16.5
Corn	2-oz. piece	15.0

Food and Description	*Measure or Quantity*	*Carbohydrates (grams)*
FROOT LOOPS, cereal (Kellogg's)	1 cup	25.0
FROSTS (Libby's):		
Dry	.5-oz.	14.0
Liquid:		
Banana	7 fl. oz.	25.0
Orange or strawberry	8 fl. oz.	29.0
Strawberry	8 fl. oz.	21.0
FROZEN DESSERT, dietetic:		
(Baskin-Robbins) *Special Diet*	1 scoop (2½ fl. oz.)	16.8
Good Humor:		
Bar, vanilla with chocolate icing	2½-fl.-oz. bar	12.0
Cup, vanilla & chocolate	5-fl.-oz. cup	17.0
(SugarLo) all flavors	¼ pt.	14.0
FRUIT BITS, dried (Sun-Maid)	1 oz.	21.0
FRUIT COCKTAIL:		
Canned, regular pack, solids & liq.:		
(Del Monte) regular or chunky	½ cup	23.0
(Libby's)	½ cup	24.7
Canned, dietetic or low calorie, solids & liq.:		
(Del Monte) Lite	½ cup	14.0
(Diet Delight):		
Syrup pack	½ cup	14.0
Water pack	½ cup	10.0
(Featherweight):		
Juice pack	½ cup	12.0
Water pack	½ cup	10.0
(Libby's) water pack	½ cup	13.0
(S&W) *Nutradiet,* white or blue label	½ cup	10.0
****FRUIT COUNTRY*** (Comstock):		
Apple	¼ of pkg.	36.0
Cherry or peach	¼ of pkg.	38.0
FRUIT CUP (Del Monte):		
Mixed fruits	5-oz. container	26.7
Peaches, diced	5-oz. container	27.8
FRUIT & FIBER CEREAL (Post):		
Apple & cinnamon	½ cup	22.3
Dates, raisins & walnuts	½ cup	21.3
FRUIT JUICE, canned (Sun-Maid), purple	6 fl. oz.	25.0
FRUIT, MIXED:		
Canned (Del Monte) Lite, chunky	½ cup	14.0
Dried (Sun-Maid/Sunsweet)	2-oz.	39.0
Frozen (Birds Eye) quick thaw	5-oz. serving	35.0

Food and Description	*Measure or Quantity*	*Carbohydrates (grams)*
FRUIT PUNCH:		
Canned:		
Capri-Sun	6¾ fl. oz.	25.9
(Hi-C)	6 fl. oz.	23.0
(Lincoln) party	6 fl. oz.	25.0
Chilled:		
Five Alive (Snow Crop)	6 fl. oz.	22.7
(Minute Maid)	6 fl. oz.	23.0
*Frozen, *Five Alive* (Snow Crop)	6 fl. oz.	22.7
*Mix:		
Regular (Hi-C)	6 fl. oz.	18.0
Dietetic, *Crystal Light*	6 fl. oz.	.1
FRUIT ROLL-UPS (Betty Crocker)	1 piece	12.0
FRUIT SALAD:		
Canned, regular pack:		
(Del Monte) fruits for salad, regular	½ cup	22.0
(Libby's)	½ cup	24.0
Canned, dietetic or low calorie:		
(Diet Delight) juice pack	½ cup	16.0
(S&W) *Nutradiet* white or blue label	½ cup	11.0
FRUIT SQUARES, frozen (Pepperidge Farm):		
Apple	2½-oz. piece	27.0
Blueberry or cherry	2½-oz. piece	29.0
FUDGSICLE (Popsicle Industries)	2½-fl.-oz. bar	23.0

G

Food and Description	*Measure or Quantity*	*Carbohydrates (grams)*
GARLIC:		
Whole	2 oz.	15.4
Flakes (Gilroy)	1 tsp.	2.6
Powder (French's)	1 tsp.	2.0
Salt (French's)	1 tsp.	1.0
GELFILTE FISH, canned:		
(Mother's):		
Jellied, old world	4-oz. serving	7.0
Jellied, white fish & pike	4-oz. serving	4.0
(Rokeach):		
Jellied, whitefish & pike	4-oz. serving	4.0
Old Vienna	4-oz. serving	8.0
GELATIN, dry, *Carmel Kosher*	7-gram envelope	0.
GELATIN DESSERT, canned, dietetic (Dia-Mel; Louis Sherry)	4-oz. serving	Tr.
***GELATIN DESSERT MIX:**		
Regular:		
Carmel Kosher, all flavors	½ cup	20.0
(Jell-O) all flavors	½ cup	18.6
Dietetic:		
Carmel Kosher	½ cup	0.
(D-Zerta) all flavors	½ cup	.1
(Estee) all flavors	½ cup	Tr.
(Featherweight) artificially sweetened	½ cup	0.
(Jell-O) sugar free	½ cup	.1
GELATIN, DRINKING (Knox) orange	1 envelope	10.0
GERMAN STYLE DINNER, frozen (Swanson) *TV Brand*	11¾-oz. dinner	36.0
GIN, SLOE:		
(DeKuyper)	1 fl. oz.	5.2
(Mr. Boston)	1 fl. oz.	4.7
GINGER, powder (French's)	1 tsp.	1.2

Food and Description	*Measure or Quantity*	*Carbohydrates (grams)*
***GINGERBREAD MIX:**		
(Betty Crocker)	1/9 of cake	35.0
(Dromedary)	2″ × 2″ square	20.0
(Pillsbury)	3″ square	36.0
***GOLDEN GRAHAMS*, cereal**		
(General Mills)	¾ cup	24.0
GOOD HUMOR (See ICE CREAM)		
GOOD N' PUDDIN		
(Popsicle Industries) all flavors	2¼-fl.-oz. bar	27.0
GOOSE, roasted, meat & skin	4 oz.	0.
***GRAHAM CRACKOS*, cereal**		
(Kellogg's)	1 cup	24.0
GRANOLA BARS, *Nature Valley:*		
Almond, oats'n honey or		
peanut butter	1 bar	16.0
Coconut or peanut	1 bar	15.0
***GRANOLA BAR MIX,** chewy,		
Nature Valley, Bake-A-Bar	1 bar	16.0
GRANOLA CEREAL:		
Nature Valley	⅓ cup	19.0
Sun Country:		
With almonds	½ cup	34.1
With raisins	½ cup	36.9
GRANOLA CLUSTERS,		
Nature Valley:		
Almond	1 piece	27.0
Caramel & raisin	1 piece	28.0
GRANOLA & FRUIT BAR,		
Nature Valley	1 bar	25.0
GRANOLA SNACK, *Nature Valley:*		
Cinnamon or honey nut	1 pouch	19.0
Peanut butter	1 pouch	17.0
GRAPE:		
American, ripe (slipskin)	3½ oz.	9.9
Canned, dietetic (Featherweight)		
light, seedless, water pack	½ cup	13.0
GRAPE DRINK:		
Canned:		
Capri Sun	6¾ fl. oz.	26.3
(Hi-C)	6 fl. oz.	22.0
(Welchade)	6 fl. oz.	23.0
*Frozen (Welchade)	6 fl. oz.	23.0
*Mix (Hi-C)	6 fl. oz.	17.0
GRAPEFRUIT:		
Pink & red:		
Seeded type	½ med. grapefruit	11.9

Food and Description	*Measure or Quantity*	*Carbohydrates (grams)*
Seedless type	½ med. grapefruit	12.8
White:		
Seeded type	½ med. grapefruit	11.7
Seedless type	½ med. grapefruit	11.9
Canned, regular pack (Del Monte) in syrup	½ cup	17.5
Canned, dietetic pack, solids & liq.:		
(Del Monte) sections	½ cup	10.4
(Diet Delight) sections	½ cup	11.0
(Featherweight) sections, juice pack	½ cup	9.0
(S&W) *Nutradiet*, blue label	½ cup	9.0
GRAPEFRUIT DRINK, canned (Lincoln)	6 fl. oz.	25.0
GRAPEFRUIT JUICE:		
Fresh, pink, red or white	½ cup	10.8
Canned, sweetened (Del Monte)	6 fl. oz.	20.8
Canned, unsweetened:		
(Del Monte)	6 fl. oz.	17.0
(Ocean Spray)	6 fl. oz.	16.2
(Texsun)	6 fl. oz.	18.0
Chilled (Minute Maid)	6 fl. oz.	18.1
GRAPEFRUIT JUICE COCKTAIL, canned (Ocean Spray) pink	6 fl. oz.	20.0
GRAPEFRUIT-ORANGE JUICE COCKTAIL, canned, *Musselman's*	6 fl. oz.	17.2
GRAPE JELLY:		
Sweetened:		
(Smucker's)	1 T.	13.5
(Welch's)	1 T.	13.5
Dietetic:		
(Dia-Mel)	1 T.	0.
(Featherweight) calorie reduced	1 T.	4.0
(Louis Sherry)	1 T.	0.
(Welch's)	1 T.	6.2
GRAPE JUICE:		
Canned, unsweetened:		
(Seneca Foods)	6 fl. oz.	30.0
(Welch's)	6 fl. oz.	30.0
*Frozen:		
(Minute Maid)	6 fl. oz.	13.3
(Welch's)	6 fl. oz.	25.0
GRAPE JUICE DRINK, chilled (Welch's)	6 fl. oz.	27.0
GRAPE NUTS, cereal (Post):		
Regular	¼ cup	23.3

Food and Description	Measure or Quantity	Carbohydrates (grams)
Flakes	⅞ cup	23.2
GRAVY, CANNED:		
Au jus (Franco-American)	2-oz. serving	2.0
Beef (Franco-American)	2-oz. serving	3.0
Brown:		
(Franco-American) with onion	2-oz. serving	4.0
(Howard Johnson's)	½ cup	4.9
Ready Gravy	¼ cup	7.5
Chicken (Franco-American) regular or giblet	2-oz. serving	3.0
Mushroom (Franco-American)	2-oz. serving	3.0
Turkey:		
(Franco-American)	2-oz. serving	3.0
(Howard Johnson's) giblet	½ cup	5.5
GRAVYMASTER	1 tsp.	2.4
GRAVY WITH MEAT OR TURKEY:		
Canned (Morton House) sliced turkey	6¼-oz. serving	7.0
Frozen:		
(Banquet):		
Giblet gravy & sliced turkey, *Cookin' Bag*	5-oz. pkg.	4.0
Sliced beef, *Buffet Supper*	2-lb. pkg.	24.0
(Morton) gravy & salisbury steak	2-lb. pkg.	52.0
(Swanson) sliced beef with whipped potatoes, *TV Brand*	8-oz. entree	19.0
GRAVY MIX:		
Regular		
Au jus:		
*(Durkee)	½ cup	3.2
*(French's) *Gravy Makins*	½ cup	1.0
Brown:		
*(Durkee):		
Regular	½ cup	5.0
With mushrooms	½ cup	5.5
*(French's) *Gravy Makins*	½ cup	6.0
(McCormick)	.85-oz. pkg.	12.8
*(Pillsbury)	½ cup	6.0
*(Spatini)	1 oz.	2.0
Chicken:		
(Durkee):		
Regular	½ cup	7.0
Roastin' Bag	1½-oz. pkg.	24.0
(McCormick)	.85-oz. pkg.	13.4
*(Pillsbury)	½ cup	8.0

Food and Description	*Measure or Quantity*	*Carbohydrates (grams)*
Home style:		
*(Durkee)	½ cup	22.0
*(Pillsbury)	½ cup	6.0
Meatloaf (Durkee) *Roastin' Bag*	1.5-oz. pkg.	18.0
Mushroom:		
*(Durkee)	½ cup	22.0
*(French's) *Gravy Makins*	½ cup	6.0
Onion:		
*(Durkee)	½ cup	7.5
*(French's) *Gravy Makins*	½ cup	8.0
(McCormick)	.84-oz. pkg.	9.8
Pork:		
*(Durkee)	½ cup	7.0
*(French's) *Gravy Makins*	½ cup	6.0
Turkey:		
*(Durkee)	½ cup	7.0
*(French's) *Gravy Makins*	½ cup	8.0
*Dietetic (Weight Watchers):		
Brown	½ cup	1.0
Brown, with mushroom or onion	½ cup	2.0
GREENS, MIXED, canned (Sunshine) solids & liq.	½ cup	2.7
GRENADINE (Garnier) no alcohol	1 fl. oz.	26.0
GUAVA, flesh only	1 guava	11.7
GUAVA NECTAR (Libby's)	6 fl. oz.	17.0

H

Food and Description	*Measure or Quantity*	*Carbohydrates (grams)*
HADDOCK:		
Fried, breaded	4″ × 3″ × ½″ fillet	5.8
Frozen:		
(Banquet)	8¾-oz. dinner	45.4
(Mrs. Paul's) breaded & fried	2-oz. fillet	10.5
(Swanson) filet almondine	7½-oz. entree	9.0
(Van de Kamp's) batter dipped, French fried	2-oz. piece	8.0
Smoked	4-oz. serving	0.
HALIBUT:		
Broiled	4″ × 3 × ½″ steak	0.
Frozen (Van de Kamp's) batter dipped, French fried	½ of 8-oz. pkg.	17.0
HAM:		
Canned:		
(Hormel):		
Chunk	6 ¾-oz. serving	Tr.
Chopped	¼ of 12-oz. can	1.0
Patties	1 patty	0.
(Oscar Mayer) *Jubilee,* extra lean, cooked	1-oz. serving	.1
Deviled:		
(Libby's)	1 oz.	0.
(Underwood)	1 oz.	Tr.
Packaged:		
(Eckrich) cooked, sliced	1.2-oz. slice	1.0
(Hormel):		
Black or red peppered	1 slice	0.
Chopped	1 slice	0.
(Oscar Mayer):		
Chopped	1-oz. slice	.9
Cooked, smoked	1-oz. slice	0.
Jubilee, boneless:		
Sliced	8-oz. slice	0.

Food and Description	Measure or Quantity	Carbohydrates (grams)
Steak, 95% fat free	2-oz. steak	0.
HAMBURGER (See *McDONALD'S, BURGER KING, DAIRY QUEEN, WHITE CASTLE,* etc.)		
HAMBURGER MIX:		
**Hamburger Helper* (General Mills):		
Beef noodle	⅕ of pkg.	25.0
Cheeseburger macaroni	⅕ of pkg.	28.0
Lasagna or pizza dish	⅕ of pkg.	33.0
Potatoes au gratin	⅕ of pkg.	27.0
Rice Oriental	⅕ of pkg.	35.0
Stew	⅕ of pkg.	23.0
Make a Better Burger (Lipton) mildly seasoned or onion	⅕ of pkg.	5.0
HAMBURGER SEASONING MIX:		
*(Durkee)	1 cup	7.5
(French's)	1-oz. pkg.	20.0
HAM & CHEESE packaged:		
(Eckrich)	1-oz. slice	1.0
(Hormel) beef	1 slice	0.
(Oscar Mayer)	1-oz. serving	.6
HAM DINNER, frozen:		
(Banquet) American Favorites	10-oz. dinner	61.0
(Morton)	10-oz. dinner	57.0
HAM SALAD, canned (Carnation)	¼ of 7 ½-oz. can	4.0
HAM SALAD SPREAD (Oscar Mayer)	1 oz.	3.0
HEADCHEESE (Oscar Mayer)	1-oz. serving	0.
HERRING, canned (Vita):		
Cocktail, drained	8-oz. jar	24.8
In cream sauce	8-oz. jar	18.1
Tastee Bits, drained	8-oz. jar	24.7
HERRING, SMOKED, kippered	4-oz. serving	0.
HICKORY NUT, shelled	1 oz.	3.6
HO-HO (Hostess)	1-oz. piece	17.0
HOMINY GRITS:		
Dry:		
(Albers) quick	1 ½ oz.	33.0
(Aunt Jemima) regular or quick	3 T.	22.5
(Quaker):		
Regular or quick	3 T.	22.5
Instant:		
Regular	.8-oz. packet	17.7
With imitation bacon or ham	1-oz. packet	21.6

Food and Description	*Measure or Quantity*	*Carbohydrates (grams)*
Cooked	1 cup	27.0
HONEY, strained	1 T.	16.5
HONEYCOMB, cereal (Post)		
regular	1 ⅓ cups	25.3
HONEYDEW	2″ × 7″ wedge	7.2
HONEY SMACKS, cereal (Kellogg's)	¾ cup	25.0
HORSERADISH:		
Raw, pared	1 oz.	5.6
Prepared (Gold's)	1 oz.	.4
HOSTESS O'S (Hostess)	2¼-oz. piece	33.0

I

Food and Description	Measure or Quantity	Carbohydrates (grams)
ICE CREAM (Listed by type, such as sandwich or *Whammy*, or by flavor—see also FROZEN DESSERT):		
Bar (Good Humor) vanilla, chocolate coated	3 fl.-oz. piece	16.0
Butter pecan:		
(Breyer's)	¼ pt.	15.0
(Good Humor) bulk	4 fl. oz.	14.0
Cherry, black (Good Humor) bulk	4 fl. oz.	14.0
Chocolate:		
(Baskin-Robbins):		
Regular	1 scoop (2 ½ fl. oz.)	20.4
Fudge	1 scoop (2 ½ fl. oz.)	21.3
(Good Humor) bulk	4 fl. oz.	15.0
(Howard Johnson's)	½ cup	25.5
Chocolate chip (Good Humor)	4 fl. oz.	15.0
Chocolate chip cookie (Good Humor)	1 sandwich (4 fl. oz.)	59.0
Chocolate eclair (Good Humor) bar	3-fl.-oz. piece	24.0
Coffee (Breyer's)	¼ pt.	15.0
Eskimo Pie, vanilla with chocolate coating	3-fl.-oz. bar	15.0
Eskimo Thin Mint, with chocolate coating	2-fl.-oz. bar	11.0
Fudge royal (Good Humor) bulk	4 fl. oz.	14.0
Peach (Breyer's)	¼ pt.	18.0
Pralines'N Cream (Baskin-Robbins)	1 scoop (2 ½ fl. oz.)	23.7
Sandwich (Good Humor)	2 ½-oz. piece	28.0
Strawberry:		
(Baskin-Robbins)	1 scoop (2 ½ fl. oz.)	15.6

Food and Description	*Measure or Quantity*	*Carbohydrates (grams)*
(Good Humor) bulk	4 fl. oz.	15.0
(Howard Johnson's)	½ cup	23.2
Toasted almond bar (Good Humor)	3-fl.-oz. piece	28.0
Toasted caramel bar (Good Humor)	3-fl.-oz. bar	21.0
Toffee fudge swirl (Good Humor) bulk	4 fl. oz.	18.0
Vanilla:		
(Baskin-Robbins) regular	1 scoop (2 ½ fl. oz.)	15.6
(Good Humor) bulk	4 fl. oz.	14.0
(Meadow Gold)	½ cup	16.0
Vanilla-chocolate-strawberry (Good Humor)	4 fl. oz.	14.0
Vanilla fudge swirl (Good Humor) bulk	4 fl. oz.	15.0
Whammy (Good Humor):		
Assorted	1.6-fl-oz. piece	9.0
Chip crunch bar	3-fl.-oz. piece	16.0
ICE CREAM CONE, cone only (Comet):		
Regular	1 piece	4.0
Rolled sugar	1 piece	9.0
ICE CREAM CUP, cup only (Comet)	1 cup	4.0
***ICE CREAM MIX** (Salada) any flavor	1 cup	32.0
ICE MILK:		
Hardened	¼ pt.	14.6
Soft-serve	¼ pt.	19.6
(Meadow Gold) vanilla, 4% fat	¼ pt.	17.0
ITALIAN DINNER, frozen (Banquet)	12-oz. dinner	446

J

Food and Description	*Measure or Quantity*	*Carbohydrates (grams)*
JELL-O FRUIT & CREAM BAR:		
Blueberry	1 bar	10.6
Peach, raspberry or strawberry	1 bar	10.9
JELL-O GELATIN POPS:		
Cherry, grape, orange or strawberry	1 piece	8.5
Raspberry	1 piece	7.7
JELL-O PUDDING POPS:		
Banana, butterscotch or vanilla	2-oz. piece	15.6
Chocolate or chocolate fudge	2-oz. piece	15.5
JELLY, sweetened		
(See individual flavors)		
JERUSALEM ARTICHOKE, pared	4 oz.	18.9
JOHANNISBERG RIESLING WINE		
(Inglenook)	3 fl. oz.	.9

K

Food and Description	*Measure or Quantity*	*Carbohydrates (grams)*
KABOOM, cereal (General Mills)	1 cup	23.0
KALE:		
Boiled, leaves only	4 oz.	6.9
Canned (Sunshine) chopped, solids & liq.	½ cup	2.8
Frozen, chopped:		
(Birds Eye)	⅓ of pkg.	4.6
(McKenzie)	3 ⅓ oz.	5.0
KARO SYRUP (See SYRUP)		
KEFIR (Alta-Dena Dairy):		
Plain	1 cup	13.0
Flavored	1 cup	24.0
KIDNEY:		
Beef, braised	4 oz.	.9
Calf, raw	4 oz.	.1
Lamb, raw	4 oz.	1.0
KIELBASA (See SAUSAGE, Polish-style)		
KING VITAMAN, cereal (Quaker)	1 ¼ cups	23.2
KIRSCH, liqueur (Garnier)	1 fl. oz.	8.8
KIX, cereal (General Mills)	1 ½ cups	24.0
KNOCKWURST	1 oz.	.6
****KOOL AID*** (General Foods):		
Unsweetened (sugar to be added)	8 fl. oz.	25.0
Pre-sweetened, with sugar:		
Apple or sunshine punch	8 fl. oz.	24.5
Cherry, grape or orange	8 fl. oz.	22.8
Tropical punch	8 fl. oz.	25.2
Pre-sweetened, sugar free:		
Cherry or grape	8 fl. oz.	.1
Sunshine or tropical punches	8 fl. oz.	.3
KUMQUAT, flesh & skin	4 oz.	19.4

L

Food and Description	Measure or Quantity	Carbohydrates (grams)
LAMB	Any quantity	0.
LASAGNA:		
Canned (Hormel) *Short Orders*	7 ½-oz. can	25.0
Frozen:		
(Green Giant):		
Bake:		
Regular, with meat sauce	12-oz. entree	44.0
Chicken	12-oz. entree	47.0
Spinach	12-oz. entree	41.0
Boil'N Bag	9 ½-oz. entree	42.0
(Stouffer's):		
Regular	10 ½-oz. serving	36.0
Lean Cuisine, zucchini	11-oz. serving	28.0
(Swanson):		
Regular, with meat in tomato sauce	13 ¼-oz. entree	45.0
Hungry Man, with meat	17 ¾-oz. dinner	90.0
(Van de Kamp's) beef & mushroom	11-oz. serving	30.0
(Weight Watchers), regular	12-oz. meal	38.0
LEEKS	4 oz.	12.7
LEMON:		
Whole	2 ⅛" lemon	11.7
Peeled	2 ⅛" lemon	6.1
LEMONADE:		
Canned:		
Capri Sun	6 ¾ fl. oz.	23.3
Country Time	6 fl. oz.	22.9
Chilled (Minute Maid) regular or pink	6 fl. oz.	18.0
*Frozen:		
Country Time, regular or pink	6 fl. oz.	24.0
Minute Maid	6 fl. oz.	19.6
*Mix, regular:		

Food and Description	*Measure or Quantity*	*Carbohydrates (grams)*
Country Time, regular or pink	6 fl. oz.	15.6
(Hi-C)	6 fl. oz.	19.0
*Mix, dietetic, *Crystal Light*	6 fl. oz.	.2
LEMON JUICE:		
Canned, *ReaLemon*	1 T.	1.1
*Frozen (Minute Maid) un-sweetened	1 fl. oz.	2.2
***LEMON-LIMEADE,** mix, *Crystal Light*	6 fl. oz.	Tr.
LEMON PEEL, candied	1 oz.	22.9
LEMON-PEPPER SEASONING (French's)	1 tsp.	1.0
LENTIL, cooked, drained	½ cup	19.5
LETTUCE:		
Bibb or Boston	4" head	4.1
Cos or Romaine, shredded or broken into pieces	½ cup	8.0
Grand Rapids, Salad Bowl or Simpson	2 large leaves	1.8
Iceberg or New York	1 lb.	12.5
LIFE, cereal (Quaker) regular or cinnamon	⅔ cup	19.7
LIL' ANGELS (Hostess)	1-oz. piece	14.0
LIME, peeled	2" dia.	4.9
***LIMEADE,** frozen (Minute Maid)	6 fl. oz.	20.1
LIME JUICE, *ReaLime*	1 T.	5.0
LIVER:		
Beef:		
Fried	6½" × 2⅜" × ⅜" slice	4.5
Cooked (Swift)	3.2-oz. serving	3.1
Calf, fried	6½" × 2⅛" × ⅜" slice	3.4
Chicken, simmered	2" × 2" × ⅝" piece	.8
LIVERWURST SPREAD (Underwood)	½ of 4¾-oz. can	3.0
LOBSTER:		
Cooked, meat only	1 cup	.4
Canned, meat only	4-oz. serving	.3
Frozen, South African lobster tail:		
3 in 8-oz. pkg.	1 piece	.2
4 in 8-oz. pkg.	1 piece	.1
5 in 8-oz. pkg.	1 piece	Tr.
LOBSTER NEWBURG	1 cup	12.8
LONG ISLAND TEA COCKTAIL (Mr. Boston) 12½% alcohol	3 fl. oz.	9.0
LUCKY CHARMS, cereal (General Mills)	1 cup	24.0

Food and Description	*Measure or Quantity*	*Carbohydrates (grams)*
LUNCHEON MEAT (See also individual listings such as BOLOGNA, HAM, etc.):		
All meat (Oscar Mayer)	1-oz. slice	.4
Banquet loaf (Eckrich)	¾-oz. slice	1.0
Bar-B-Que Loaf (Oscar Mayer) 90% fat free	1-oz. slice	1.4
Beef, jellied (Hormel) loaf	1 slice	0
Gourmet loaf (Eckrich)	1-oz. slice	2.0
Ham and cheese (See HAM & CHEESE)		
Ham roll sausage (Oscar Mayer)	1-oz. slice	.6
Honey loaf:		
(Eckrich)	1-oz. slice	3.0
(Oscar Mayer) 95% fat free	1-oz. slice	1.1
Iowa brand (Hormel)	1 slice	0.
Liver cheese (Oscar Mayer)	1.3-oz. slice	.6
Liver loaf (Hormel)	1-oz. slice	6.5
Luxury loaf (Oscar Mayer) 95% fat free	1-oz. slice	1.5
Macaroni-cheese loaf (Eckrich)	1-oz. slice	3.0
Meat loaf	1-oz. serving	.9
New England brand sliced sausage:		
(Eckrich)	1-oz. slice	1.0
(Oscar Mayer) 92% fat free	.8-oz. slice	.3
Old fashioned loaf (Oscar Mayer)	1-oz. slice	2.3
Olive loaf:		
(Eckrich)	1-oz. slice	2.0
(Hormel)	1-oz. slice	1.5
Peppered loaf:		
(Eckrich)	1-oz. slice	1.0
(Oscar Mayer) 93% fat free	1-oz. slice	1.3
Pickle loaf:		
(Eckrich)	1-oz. slice	2.0
(Hormel)	1 slice	1.5
Pickle & pimiento (Oscar Mayer)	1-oz. slice	3.0
Picnic loaf (Oscar Mayer)	1-oz. slice	1.6
Spiced (Hormel)	1 slice	.5

M

Food and Description	Measure or Quantity	Carbohydrates (grams)
MACADAMIA NUT		
(Royal Hawaiian)	1 oz.	4.5
MACARONI:		
Cooked:		
8–10 minutes, firm	1 cup	39.1
14–20 minutes, tender	1 cup	32.2
Canned (Franco-American):		
Beefy Mac	7½-oz. can	30.0
PizzOs	7½-oz. can	35.0
Frozen:		
(Banquet) & beef:		
Regular	12-oz. dinner	55.1
Buffet Supper	2-lb. pkg.	106.4
(Morton)	10-oz. dinner	46.0
(Stouffer's) with tomatoes	5¾-oz. serving	20.0
MACARONI & CHEESE:		
Canned:		
(Franco-American) regular or elbow	7⅜-oz. serving	24.0
(Hormel) *Short Orders*	7½-oz. can	23.0
Frozen:		
(Banquet):		
Buffet Supper	2-lb. pkg.	148.0
Casserole	8-oz. pkg.	36.0
(Green Giant) *Boil 'N Bag*	9-oz. entree	290.0
(Morton) dinner	11-oz. dinner	54.0
(Swanson):		
Regular	12-oz. dinner	43.0
TV Brand	12¼-oz. dinner	48.0
Mix:		
(Golden Grain) deluxe	¼ of 7¼-oz. pkg.	38.1
(Lipton)	½ cup	25.0
*(Prince)	¾ cup	34.6

Food and Description	*Measure or Quantity*	*Carbohydrates (grams)*
MACARONI & CHEESE PIE, frozen (Swanson)	7-oz. pie	25.0
MACARONI SALAD, canned (Nalley's)	4-oz. serving	15.9
MACKEREL, Atlantic, broiled, with fat	8½" × 2½" × ½" fillet	0.
MALTED MILK MIX (Carnation):		
Chocolate	3 heaping tsps.	18.4
Natural	3 heaping tsps.	15.8
MALT LIQUOR, *Champale,* regular	12 fl. oz.	12.2
MALT-O-MEAL, cereal	1 T.	7.3
MANDARIN ORANGE (See TANGERINE)		
MANGO, fresh	1 med. mango	22.5
MANGO NECTAR (Libby's)	6 fl. oz.	14.0
MANHATTAN COCKTAIL (Mr. Boston) 20% alcohol	3 fl. oz.	6.3
MAPLE SYRUP (See SYRUP, Maple)		
MARGARINE:		
Regular	1 pat (1" × 1.3" × 1", 5 grams)	Tr.
(Mazola)	1 T.	.2
(Promise) regular, soft or squeeze	1 T.	Tr.
MARGARINE, IMITATION OR DIETETIC:		
(Imperial) diet or light	1 T.	Tr.
(Mazola)	1 T.	Tr.
MARGARINE, WHIPPED (Blue Bonnet; Miracle; Parkay)	1 T.	Tr.
MARGARITA COCKTAIL, (Mr. Boston):		
Regular	3 fl. oz.	10.8
Strawberry	3 fl. oz.	18.9
MARINADE MIX:		
Chicken (Adolph's)	1-oz. packet	14.4
Meat:		
(Adolph's)	.8-oz. pkg.	8.5
(French's)	1-oz. pkg.	16.5
(Kikkoman)	1-oz. pkg.	12.5
MARJORAM (French's)	1 tsp.	.8
MARMALADE:		
Sweetened (Keiller):	1 T.	14.9
Dietetic:		
(Dia-Mel; Louis Sherry)	1 T.	0.
(Featherweight)	1 T.	4.0
(S&W) *Nutradiet,* red label	1 T.	3.0

Food and Description	*Measure or Quantity*	*Carbohydrates (grams)*
MARSHMALLOW FLUFF	1 heaping tsp.	14.4
MARSHMALLOW KRISPIES, cereal		
(Kellogg's)	1¼ cups	33.0
MARTINI COCKTAIL (Mr. Boston):		
Gin, extra dry, 20% alcohol	3 fl. oz.	0.
Vodka, 20% alcohol	3 fl. oz.	0.
MASA HARINA (Quaker)	⅓ cup	27.4
MASA TRIGO (Quaker)	⅓ cup	24.7
MATZO (Horowitz-Margareten)		
regular	1 matzo	28.1
MAYONNAISE:		
Real, *Hellmann's* (Best Foods)	1 T.	.1
Imitation or dietetic:		
(Diet Delight) *Mayo-Lite*	1 T.	0.
(Weight Watchers)	1 T.	1.0
MAYPO, cereal:		
30-second	¼ cup	16.4
Vermont style	¼ cup	22.0
McDONALD'S:		
Big Mac	1 hamburger	40.6
Cheeseburger	1 cheeseburger	29.8
Chicken McNuggets	1 serving (3.9 oz.)	15.4
Chicken McNuggets Sauce:		
Barbecue	1.1 oz.	13.7
Honey	.5 oz.	12.4
Sweet & Sour	1.1 oz.	15.0
Cookies:		
Chocolate chip	1 package	44.8
McDonaldland	1 package	48.7
Egg McMuffin	1 serving	31.0
Egg, scrambled	1 serving	2.5
English muffin, with butter	1 muffin	29.5
Filet-O-Fish	1 sandwich	37.4
Grapefruit juice	6 fl. oz.	17.9
Hamburger	1 hamburger	29.5
Hot cakes with butter & syrup	1 serving	93.9
Orange juice	6 fl. oz.	19.6
Pie:		
Apple	1 pie	29.3
Cherry	1 pie	32.1
Potato:		
Fried	1 regular order	26.1
Hash browns	1 order	14.0
Quarter Pounder:		
Regular	1 hamburger	32.7
With cheese	1 hamburger	32.2

Food and Description	*Measure or Quantity*	*Carbohydrates (grams)*
Sausage, pork	1 serving	.6
Shake:		
Chocolate	1 serving	65.5
Strawberry	1 serving	62.1
Vanilla	1 serving	59.6
Sundae:		
Caramel	1 serving	52.5
Hot fudge or strawberry	1 serving	46.2
MEATBALL DINNER or ENTREE, frozen:		
(Green Giant)	9.4-oz. entree	57.0
(Swanson) *TV Brand*	9¼-oz. entree	21.0
MEATBALL SEASONING MIX:		
*(Durkee) Italian style	1 cup	4.5
(French's)	1.5-oz. pkg.	28.0
MEATBALL STEW:		
Canned:		
Dinty Moore (Hormel)	7½-oz. serving	15.1
(Libby's)	8-oz. serving	24.3
Frozen (Stouffer's) *Lean Cuisine*	10-oz. pkg.	21.0
MEATBALLS, SWEDISH, frozen (Stouffer's) with noodles	11-oz. pkg.	33.0
MEAT LOAF DINNER, frozen:		
(Banquet):		
American Favorite	11-oz. dinner	30.0
Extra Helping	19-oz. dinner	80.0
(Morton)	11-oz. dinner	28.0
(Swanson) *TV Brand,* with tomato sauce & whipped potatoes	9-oz. entree	28.0
MEAT LOAF SEASONING MIX (French's)	1.5-oz. pkg.	40.0
MEAT, POTTED (Libby's)	1-oz. serving	0.
MEAT TENDERIZER (Adolph's)	1 tsp.	Tr.
MELBA TOAST, salted (Old London):		
Garlic, onion or white rounds	1 piece	1.8
Pumpernickel, rye, wheat or white	1 piece	3.4
MELON BALL, in syrup, frozen	½ cup	18.2
MERLOT WINE (Louis M. Martini)	3 fl. oz.	.2
MEXICAN DINNER, frozen:		
(Banquet) combination	12-oz. dinner	72.0
(Swanson) *TV Brand*	16-oz. dinner	66.0
(Van de Kamp's)	11½-oz. dinner	43.0
MILK BREAK BARS (Pillsbury):		
Chocolate	1 bar	22.0
Natural or peanut butter	1 bar	21.0

Food and Description	*Measure or Quantity*	*Carbohydrates (grams)*
MILK, CONDENSED, (Carnation)	1 fl. oz.	20.8
***MILK, DRY,** non-fat, instant (Alba; Carnation, Pet; *Sanalac*)	1 cup	11.0
MILK, EVAPORATED:		
Regular:		
(Carnation)	1 fl. oz.	3.1
(Pet)	½ cup	12.5
Filled (Dairymate)	½ cup	12.0
Low fat (Carnation)	1 fl. oz.	3.0
Skimmed, *Pet 99*	½ cup	14.0
MILK, FRESH:		
Buttermilk (Friendship)	8 fl. oz.	12.0
Chocolate (Dairylea)	8 fl. oz.	24.0
Skim (Dairylea; Meadow Gold)	1 cup	11.0
Whole (Dairylea; Meadow Gold)	1 cup	11.0
MILK, GOAT, whole	1 cup	11.2
MILK, HUMAN	1 oz.	2.7
MILNOT, dairy vegetable blend	1 fl. oz.	3.1
MINERAL WATER (Schweppes)	6 fl. oz.	0.
MINI-WHEATS, cereal (Kellogg's)	1 biscuit	6.0
MINT LEAVES	½ oz.	.8
MOLASSES:		
Barbados	1 T.	13.3
Blackstrap	1 T.	10.4
Dark (Brer Rabbit)	1 T.	10.6
Light	1 T.	12.4
Medium	1 T.	11.4
Unsulphured (Grandma's)	1 T.	15.0
MORTADELLA sausage	1 oz.	.2
MOST, cereal (Kellogg's)	½ cup	22.0
MOUSSE, canned, dietetic (Featherweight) chocolate	½ cup	14.0
MUFFIN:		
Blueberry:		
(Morton) rounds	1½-oz. muffin	21.0
(Pepperidge Farm)	1.9-oz. muffin	27.0
Bran (Arnold) *Bran'nola*	2.3-oz. muffin	30.0
Corn:		
(Pepperidge Farm)	1.9-oz. muffin	27.0
(Thomas')	2-oz. muffin	25.8
English:		
(Arnold) extra crisp	2.3-oz. muffin	30.0
(Pepperidge Farm):		
Plain	2-oz. muffin	26.0
Cinnamon apple	2-oz. muffin	27.0
Wheat	2-oz. muffin	25.0

Food and Description	*Measure or Quantity*	*Carbohydrates (grams)*
Roman Meal	2.3-oz. muffin	29.8
(Thomas') regular	2-oz. muffin	25.7
(Wonder)	2-oz. muffin	26.0
Orange-cranberry (Pepperidge Farm)	2.1-oz. muffin	30.0
Plain, home recipe	1.4-oz. muffin	16.9
Raisin (Arnold)	2.5-oz. muffin	35.0
Sourdough (Wonder)	2-oz. muffin	27.0
MUFFIN MIX:		
*Apple (Betty Crocker) spiced	1 muffin	18.0
Blueberry (Betty Crocker) wild	1 muffin	120
Bran (Duncan Hines)	1/12 of pkg.	16.3
*Cherry (Betty Crocker)	1/12 of pkg.	18.0
Corn:		
*(Betty Crocker)	1 muffin	25.0
*(Dromedary)	1 muffin	20.0
MULLIGAN STEW, canned, *Dinty Moore, Short Orders* (Hormel)	7½-oz. can	14.0
MUSCATEL WINE (Gallo) 14% alcohol	3 fl. oz.	86
MUSHROOM:		
Raw, whole	½ lb.	9.7
Raw, trimmed, sliced	½ cup	1.5
Canned (Green Giant):		
Whole or sliced	2-oz. serving	2.0
Whole or sliced, in butter sauce	½ of 3 ½-oz. can	3.5
Frozen (Green Giant) whole, in butter sauce	½ cup	5.0
MUSHROOM, CHINESE, dried	1 oz.	18.9
MUSSEL, in shell	1 lb.	7.2
MUSTARD:		
Powder (French's)	1 tsp.	.3
Prepared:		
Brown (French's; Gulden's)	1 tsp.	.3
Dijon, *Grey Poupon*	1 tsp.	Tr.
Horseradish (Nalley's)	1 tsp.	.3
MUSTARD GREENS:		
Canned (Sunshine) solids & liq.	½ cup	3.2
Frozen, chopped:		
(Birds Eye)	⅓ of pkg.	3.2
(Southland)	⅓ of 16-oz. pkg.	3.0
MUSTARD SPINACH:		
Raw	1 lb.	17.7
Boiled, drained, no added salt	4-oz. serving	3.2

N

Food and Description	Measure or Quantity	Carbohydrates (grams)
NATURAL CEREAL:		
Heartland (Quaker):	¼ cup	17.9
Hot, whole wheat	⅓ cup	21.8
100% natural	¼ cup	17.4
100% with raisins & dates	¼ cup	18.0
NATURE SNACKS (Sun-Maid):		
Carob Crunch	1 oz.	16.8
Carob Peanut or Yogurt Peanut	1 ¼ oz.	18.0
Raisin Crunch or Rocky Road	1 oz.	19.7
Sesame Nut Crunch	1 oz.	14.6
NECTARINE, flesh only	4 oz.	19.4
NOODLE:		
Dry (Pennsylvania Dutch Brand) any type	1 oz.	20.0
Cooked, 1½" strips	1 cup	37.3
NOODLES & BEEF:		
Canned (Hormel) *Short Orders*	7½-oz. can	16.0
Frozen (Banquet) *Buffet Supper*	2-lb. pkg.	83.6
NOODLES & CHICKEN:		
Canned (Hormel) *Dinty Moore, Short Orders*	7½-oz. can	15.0
Frozen (Swanson) *TV Brand*	10½-oz. dinner	37.0
NOODLE, CHOW MEIN (La Choy)	½ cup	17.0
NOODLE MIX:		
*(Betty Crocker):		
Fettucini Alfredo or Romanoff	¼ of pkg.	23.0
Stroganoff	¼ of pkg.	26.0
Noodle Roni, parmesano	⅕ of 6-oz. pkg.	22.5
*(Lipton):		
Beef	½ cup	26.0
Cheese	½ cup	24.0
Chicken	½ cup	25.0
Sour cream & chive	½ cup	23.0

Food and Description	*Measure or Quantity*	*Carbohydrates (grams)*
NOODLE, RICE (La Choy)	1 oz.	21.0
NOODLE ROMANOFF, frozen (Stouffer's)	⅓ of pkg.	16.0
NUT, MIXED:		
Dry roasted:		
(Flavor House)	1 oz.	5.4
(Planters)	1 oz.	7.0
Oil roasted (Planters) with or without peanuts	1 oz.	6.0
NUTMEG (French's)	1 tsp.	.9
NUTRI-GRAIN, cereal (Kellogg's):		
Corn	½ cup	24.0
Wheat	⅔ cup	24.0
Wheat & raisin	⅔ cup	33.0
NUTRIMATO (Mott's)	6 fl. oz.	17.0

O

Food and Description	*Measure or Quantity*	*Carbohydrates (grams)*
OAT FLAKES, cereal (Post)	⅔ cup	20.6
OATMEAL:		
Dry:		
Regular:		
(Elam's) Scotch style	1 oz.	18.2
(H-O) old fashioned	1 T.	2.6
(Quaker) old fashioned	⅓ cup	18.5
Instant:		
(H-O):		
Regular, boxed	1 T.	2.6
With bran & spice	1½-oz. packet	20.0
With maple & brown sugar flavor	1½-oz. packet	31.8
(Quaker):		
Regular	1-oz. packet	18.1
Apple & cinnamon and honey & graham	1¼-oz. packet	26.0
Raisins & spice	1½-oz. packet	31.4
(3-Minute Brand)	½ cup	25.9
Quick:		
(Harvest Brand)	⅓ cup	18.1
(H-O)	½ cup	22.2
(Ralston Purina)	⅓ cup	18.0
(3-Minute Brand)	⅓ cup	18.1
Cooked, regular	1 cup	23.3
OIL, SALAD OR COOKING	Any quantity	0.
OKRA, frozen:		
(Birds Eye) whole	⅓ of pkg.	6.7
(Seabrook Farms) cut	⅓ of pkg.	6.1
(Southland) whole	⅓ of 16-oz. pkg.	7.0
OLIVE:		
Green	4 med. or 3 extra large or 2 giant	.2
Ripe, Mission	3 small or 2 large	.3

Food and Description	Measure or Quantity	Carbohydrates (grams)
OMELET, frozen (Swanson)		
TV Brand, Spanish style	7¾-oz. entree	16.0
ONION:		
Raw	2½" onion	8.7
Boiled, pearl onion	½ cup	6.0
Canned (Durkee) *O & C:*		
Boiled	¼ of 16-oz. jar.	8.0
Creamed	¼ of 15½-oz. can	65.8
Dehydrated (Gilroy) flakes	1 tsp.	1.2
Frozen:		
(Birds Eye):		
Chopped	1 oz.	2.0
Creamed	⅓ of pkg.	11.4
Whole, small	⅓ of pkg.	9.6
(Green Giant) in cheese sauce	½ cup	9.0
(Mrs. Paul's) french-fried rings	½ of 5-oz. pkg.	22.2
(Southland) chopped	⅕ of 10-oz. pkg.	5.0
ONION BOUILLON:		
(Herb-Ox)	1 cube	1.3
MBI	1 packet	2.0
ONION, GREEN	1 small onion	.9
ONION SALAD SEASONING		
(French's) instant	1 T.	3.0
ONION SALT (French's)	1 tsp.	1.0
ONION SOUP (See SOUP, Onion)		
ORANGE:		
Peeled	½ cup	15.5
Sections	4 oz.	14.4
ORANGE DRINK:		
Canned:		
Capri Sun	6 ¾-oz. can	26.1
(Hi-C)	6 fl. oz.	23.0
*Mix:		
Regular (Hi-C)	6 fl. oz.	17.0
Dietetic, *Crystal Light*	6 fl. oz.	.4
ORANGE EXTRACT (Durkee)		
imitation	1 tsp.	15.0
ORANGE-GRAPEFRUIT JUICE:		
Canned (Libby's) unsweetened	6 fl. oz.	19.0
*Frozen (Minute Maid) unsweetened	6 fl. oz.	19.1
ORANGE JUICE:		
Canned:		
(Del Monte) sweetened	6 fl. oz.	76.0
(Libby's) unsweetened	6 fl. oz.	90.0
Chilled (Minute Maid)	6 fl. oz.	19.7

Food and Description	*Measure or Quantity*	*Carbohydrates (grams)*
*Frozen:		
Bright & Early, imitation	6 fl. oz.	21.6
Orange Plus (Birds Eye)	6 fl. oz.	24.0
(Snow Crop)	6 fl. oz.	20.5
ORANGE PEEL, candied	1 oz.	22.9
ORANGE-PINEAPPLE DRINK, canned (Lincoln)	8 fl. oz.	24.0
ORANGE-PINEAPPLE JUICE, canned (Texsun)	8 fl. oz.	19.0
OVALTINE, chocolate or malt	¾ oz.	17.9
OVEN FRY (General Foods):		
Crispy crumb for pork	4.2-oz. envelope	78.0
Extra crispy for chicken	4.2-oz. envelope	76.5
OYSTER:		
Raw:		
Eastern	19–31 small or 13–19 med.	8.2
Pacific & Western	6–9 small or 4–6 med.	15.4
Canned (Bumble Bee) shelled, whole, solids & liq.	1 cup	15.4
Fried	4 oz.	21.1
OYSTER STEW, home recipe	½ cup	7.1

P

Food and Description	Measure or Quantity	Carbohydrates (grams)
PAC-MAN CEREAL (General Mills)	1 cup	25.0
***PANCAKE BATTER, FROZEN** (Aunt Jemima):		
Plain or buttermilk	4″ pancake	14.1
Blueberry	4″ pancake	13.8
PANCAKE & SAUSAGE, frozen (Swanson)	6-oz. entree	48.0
***PANCAKE & WAFFLE MIX:**		
Plain:		
(Aunt Jemima):		
Complete	4″ pancake	15.7
Original	4″ pancake	8.7
(Log Cabin):		
Complete	4″ pancake	11.2
Original	4″ pancake	8.7
(Pillsbury) *Hungry Jack:*		
Complete, bulk or packets	4″ pancake	13.0
Extra Lights	4″ pancake	10.0
Golden Blend, complete	4″ pancake	14.3
Blueberry (Pillsbury) *Hungry Jack*	4″ pancake	13.3
Buckwheat (Aunt Jemima)	4″ pancake	8.3
Buttermilk:		
(Aunt Jemima):		
Regular	4″ pancake	13.3
Complete	4″ pancake	15.3
(Pillsbury) *Hungry Jack,* complete	4″ pancake	13.0
Whole wheat (Aunt Jemima)	4″ pancake	10.7
Dietetic:		
(Dia-Mel)	3″ pancake	7.0
(Featherweight)	4″ pancake	8.0
PANCAKE & WAFFLE SYRUP (See SYRUP, Pancake & Waffle)		
PAPAYA, fresh:		
Cubed	½ cup	9.1

Food and Description	Measure or Quantity	Carbohydrates (grams)
Juice	4 oz.	18.8
PAPRIKA (French's)	1 tsp.	1.1
PARSLEY:		
Fresh, chopped	1 T.	.3
Dried (French's)	1 tsp.	.6
PASTINAS, egg	1 oz.	20.4
PASTRAMI (Eckrich) sliced	1-oz. serving	1.0
PASTRY SHEET, PUFF, frozen (Pepperidge Farm)	1 sheet	45.0
PÂTE:		
De foie gras	1 T.	.7
Liver (Hormel)	1 T.	.3
PDQ, Chocolate or strawberry	1 T.	15.0
PEA, green:		
Boiled	½ cup	9.9
Canned, regular pack, solids & liq.:		
(Del Monte) small	½ cup	9.0
(Green Giant):		
Early, with onions	½ cup	10.0
Sweet	½ cup	11.0
Sweet, with onions	½ cup	10.9
(Libby's) sweet	½ cup	11.6
Canned, dietetic pack, solids & liq.:		
(Del Monte) No Salt Added	½ cup	11.0
(Diet Delight)	½ cup	8.0
(Featherweight) sweet	½ cup	12.0
Frozen:		
(Birds Eye):		
Regular	⅓ of pkg.	13.3
In butter sauce	⅓ of pkg.	12.6
In cream sauce	⅓ of pkg.	14.3
(Green Giant):		
Creamed	½ cup	12.0
Early & sweet in butter sauce	½ cup	10.0
Sweet, *Harvest Fresh*	½ cup	14.0
PEA & CARROT:		
Canned, regular pack, solids & liq.:		
(Del Monte)	½ cup	10.0
(Libby's)	½ cup	10.3
Canned, dietetic pack, solids & liq.:		
(Diet Delight)	½ cup	6.0
(S&W) *Nutradiet*	½ cup	7.0
Frozen:		
(Birds Eye)	⅓ of pkg.	11.2
(McKenzie)	3.3-oz. serving	11.0

Food and Description	*Measure or Quantity*	*Carbohydrates (grams)*
PEA, CROWDER, frozen		
(Southland)	⅓ of 16-oz. pkg.	21.0
PEA POD:		
Boiled, drained solids	4 oz.	10.8
Frozen (La Choy)	6-oz. pkg.	12.0
PEACH:		
Fresh, with thin skin	2″ peach	9.6
Fresh, slices	½ cup	8.2
Canned, regular pack, solids & liq.:		
(Del Monte) Cling:		
Halves & slices	½ cup	22.0
Spiced	3 ½-oz. serving	20.0
(Libby's) heavy syrup:		
Halves	½ cup	25.4
Sliced	½ cup	24.7
Canned, dietetic pack, solids & liq.:		
(Del Monte) Lite	½ cup	13.0
(Diet Delight) Cling:		
Juice pack	½ cup	11.0
Water pack	½ cup	8.0
Frozen (Birds Eye)	5-oz. serving	34.0
PEACH BUTTER (Smucker's)	1 T.	16.0
PEACH DRINK, canned (Hi-C):		
Canned	6 fl. oz.	23.0
*Mix	6 fl. oz.	18.0
PEACH LIQUEUR (DeKuyper)	1 fl. oz.	8.3
PEACH NECTAR, canned (Libby's)	6 fl. oz.	23.0
PEACH PRESERVE OR JAM:		
Sweetened (Smucker's)	1 T.	13.5
Dietetic:		
(Dia-Mel)	1 T.	0.
(Featherweight) artificially sweetened	1 T.	1.0
PEANUT:		
Raw, with skins	1 oz.	5.3
Dry roasted:		
(Fisher)	1 oz.	5.0
(Planters)	1 oz.	6.0
Oil roasted (Planters)	1 oz.	5.0
PEANUT BUTTER:		
Regular:		
(Elam's) natural	1 T.	2.1
(Jif) creamy	1 T.	2.7
(Peter Pan):		
Crunchy	1 T.	3.0
Smooth	1 T.	3.1

Food and Description	Measure or Quantity	Carbohydrates (grams)
(Skippy):		
Creamy	1 T.	3.0
Creamy, old fashioned	1 T.	2.8
Dietetic:		
(Featherweight) low sodium	1 T.	2.0
(Peter Pan) low sodium	1 T.	2.3
(S&W) *Nutradiet,* low sodium	1 T.	2.0
PEANUT BUTTER		
BAKING CHIPS (Reese's)	3 T. (1 oz.)	12.8
PEAR:		
Whole	3″ × 2½″ pear	25.4
Canned, regular pack, solids & liq.:		
(Del Monte) Bartlett	½ cup	22.0
(Libby's)	½ cup	25.1
Canned, dietetic pack, solids & liq.:		
(Del Monte) Lite	½ cup	14.0
(Diet Delight) juice pack	½ cup	16.0
(Featherweight) Bartlett:		
Juice pack	½ cup	15.0
Water pack	½ cup	10.0
(Libby's) water pack	½ cup	15.0
Dried (Sun-Maid)	½ cup	70.0
PEAR NECTAR, canned (Libby's)	6 fl. oz.	25.0
PEAR-PASSION FRUIT NECTAR,		
canned (Libby's)	6 fl. oz.	14.0
PEBBLES, cereal	⅞ cup	24.4
PECAN:		
Halves	6–7 pieces	1.1
Roasted, dry:		
(Fisher) salted	1 oz.	4.5
(Planters)	1 oz.	5.0
PECTIN, FRUIT:		
Certo	6-oz. pkg.	4.8
Sure-Jell	1¾-oz. pkg.	10.7
PEP, cereal (Kellogg's)	¾ cup	23.0
PEPPER:		
Black (French's)	1 tsp.	1.5
Seasoned (French's)	1 tsp.	1.0
PEPPER, CHILI, canned:		
(Del Monte):		
Green, whole	½ cup	5.0
Jalapeno or chili, whole	½ cup	6.0
Old El Paso, green,		
chopped or whole	1 oz.	1.4
(Ortega):		
Diced, strips or whole	1 oz.	1.1

Food and Description	*Measure or Quantity*	*Carbohydrates (grams)*
Jalapeno, diced or whole	1 oz.	1.7
PEPPERONI:		
(Eckrich)	1-oz. serving	1.0
(Hormel)	1-oz. serving	0.
PEPPER & ONION, frozen (Southland):		
Diced	2-oz. serving	3.0
Red & green	2-oz. serving	4.0
PEPPER STEAK, frozen (Stouffer's)	10½-oz. pkg.	35.0
PEPPER, STUFFED:		
Home recipe	2¾" × 2½" pepper with 1 ⅛ cups stuffing	31.1
Frozen:		
(Green Giant) green, baked	7-oz. serving	15.0
(Stouffer's)	7¼-oz. serving	18.0
(Weight Watchers) with veal stuffing	11 ¾-oz. meal	22.0
PEPPER, SWEET:		
Raw:		
Green:		
Whole	1 lb.	17.9
Without stem & seeds	1 med. pepper (2.6 oz.)	2.9
Red:		
Whole	1 lb.	25.8
Without stem & seeds	1 med. pepper (2.2 oz.)	2.4
Boiled, green, without salt, drained	1 med. pepper (2.6 oz.)	2.8
Frozen:		
(McKenzie)	1-oz. serving	1.0
(Southland)	2-oz. serving	3.0
PERNOD (Julius Wile)	1 fl. oz.	1.1
PERSIMMON:		
Japanese or Kaki, fresh:		
With seeds	4.4-oz. piece	20.1
Seedless	4.4-oz. piece	20.7
Native, fresh, flesh only	4-oz. serving	38.0
PHEASANT, raw, meat only	Any quantity	0.
PICKLE:		
Cucumber, fresh or bread & butter:		
(Fannings)	1.2-oz. serving	3.9
(Featherweight)	1-oz. pickle	3.0
(Nalley's) chips	1-oz. serving	6.5

Food and Description	*Measure or Quantity*	*Carbohydrates (grams)*
Dill:		
(Featherweight) low sodium, whole	1-oz. serving	1.0
(Smucker's):		
Hamburger, sliced	1 slice	0.
Polish, whole	3½" pickle	1.0
Hamburger (Nalley's) chips	1-oz. serving	.6
Kosher dill:		
(Claussen) halves or whole	2-oz. serving	1.3
(Featherweight) low sodium	1-oz. serving	1.0
(Smucker's):		
Baby	2¾-oz. long pickle	.5
Slices	1 slice	0.
Whole	2½" long pickle	1.0
Sweet:		
(Nalley's) *Nubbins*	1-oz. serving	7.9
(Smucker's):		
Candied mix	1 piece	3.3
Gherkins	2" long pickle	3.5
Whole	2½" long pickle	4.0
Sweet & sour (Claussen) slices	1 slice	.8
PIE:		
Regular, non-frozen:		
Apple:		
Home recipe, two-crust	⅙ of 9" pie	60.2
(Hostess)	4½-oz. pie	45.0
Banana, home recipe, cream or custard	⅙ of 9" pie	46.7
Berry (Hostess)	4½-oz. pie	48.0
Blackberry, home recipe, two-crust	⅙ of 9" pie	54.4
Blueberry:		
Home recipe, two-crust	⅙ of 9" pie	55.1
(Hostess)	4½-oz. pie	49.0
Boston cream, home recipe	1/12 of 8" pie	34.4
Butterscotch, home recipe, one-crust	⅙ of 9" pie	58.2
Cherry:		
Home recipe, two-crust	⅙ of 9" pie	60.7
(Hostess)	4½-oz. pie	55.0
Chocolate chiffon, home recipe	⅙ of 9" pie	61.2
Chocolate meringue, home recipe	⅙ of 9" pie	46.9
Coconut custard, home recipe	⅙ of 9" pie	37.8
Lemon (Hostess)	4½-oz. pie	53.0
Mince, home recipe, two-crust	⅙ of 9" pie	65.1
Peach (Hostess)	4½-oz. pie	53.0

Food and Description	*Measure or Quantity*	*Carbohydrates (grams)*
Pumpkin, home recipe, one-crust	⅙ of 9″ pie	37.2
Raisin, home recipe, two-crust	⅙ of 9″ pie	67.9
Strawberry (Hostess)	4½-oz. pie	56.0
Frozen:		
Apple:		
(Banquet)	⅕ of 20-oz. pie	37.0
(Morton):		
Regular	⅙ of 24-oz. pie	41.0
Great Little Desserts	8-oz. pie	88.0
(Sara Lee) regular	⅙ of 31-oz. pie	43.2
Banana cream:		
(Banquet)	⅙ of 14-oz. pie	21.0
(Morton) *Great Little Desserts*	3½-oz. pie	27.0
Blueberry:		
(Banquet)	⅙ of 20-oz. pie	40.0
(Morton) *Great Little Desserts*	8-oz. pie	86.0
Cherry:		
(Morton) regular	⅙ of 24-oz. pie	42.0
(Sara Lee)	⅙ of 31-oz. pie	48.0
Chocolate cream:		
(Banquet)	⅙ of 14-oz. pie	24.0
(Morton) *Great Little Desserts*	3½-oz. pie	29.0
Coconut (Morton)	⅙ of 14-oz. pie	17.0
Coconut cream (Banquet)	⅙ of 14-oz. pie	22.0
Coconut custard:		
(Banquet)	⅙ of 20-oz. pie	28.2
(Morton) *Great Little Desserts*	6½-oz. pie	53.0
Lemon cream (Banquet)	⅙ of 14-oz. pie	23.0
Mince:		
(Banquet)	⅙ of 20-oz. pie	38.0
(Morton)	⅙ of 24-oz. pie	46.0
Peach (Sara Lee)	⅙ of 31-oz. pie	56.2
Pumpkin:		
(Banquet)	⅙ of 20-oz. pie	29.0
(Morton)	⅙ of 24-oz. pie	36.0
Strawberry cream (Banquet)	⅙ of 14-oz. pie	22.0
PIECRUST:		
Home recipe, 9″ pie	1 crust	78.0
Frozen (Banquet) 9″ shell:		
Regular	1 crust	61.9
Deep Dish	1 crust	78.8
Refrigerated (Pillsbury)	2-crust pie shell	184.0
***PIECRUST MIX:**		
(Betty Crocker):		
Regular	1/16 of pkg.	10.0
Stick	⅛ of stick	10.0

Food and Description	*Measure or Quantity*	*Carbohydrates (grams)*
(Flako)	⅙ of 9″ pie shell	25.2
(Pillsbury) mix or stick	⅙ of 2-crust pie	25.0
PIE FILLING (See also PUDDING OR PIE FILLING):		
Apple (Comstock)	⅙ of 21-oz. can	24.0
Apple rings or slices (See APPLE, canned)		
Apricot (Comstock)	⅙ of 21-oz. can	24.0
Banana cream (Comstock)	⅙ of 21-oz. can	26.0
Blueberry (Comstock)	⅙ of 21-oz. can	26.0
Coconut cream (Comstock)	⅙ of 21-oz. can	26.0
Coconut custard, home recipe, made with egg yolk & milk	5 oz. (inc. crust)	41.3
Lemon (Comstock)	⅙ of 21-oz. can	33.0
Mincemeat (Comstock)	½ of 21-oz. can	36.0
Pumpkin (Libby's) (See also PUMPKIN, canned)	1 cup	58.0
Raisin (Comstock)	⅙ of 21-oz. can	30.0
***PIE MIX** (Betty Crocker)		
Boston cream	⅛ of pie	48.0
PIEROGIES, frozen (Mrs. Paul's)		
potato & cheese	1 pierogi	14.7
PIGS FEET, pickled	4-oz. serving	0.
PIMIENTO, canned:		
(Dromedary) drained	1-oz. serving	2.0
(Sunshine) diced or sliced solids & liq.	1 T.	.9
PINA COLADA (Mr. Boston)		
12 ½% alcohol	3 fl. oz.	34.2
PINEAPPLE:		
Fresh, diced	½ cup	10.7
Canned, regular pack, solids & liq.:		
(Del Monte) slices, medium	½ cup	12.0
(Dole):		
Juice pack, chunk, crushed or sliced	½ cup	18.0
Heavy syrup, chunk, crushed or sliced	½ cup	23.0
Canned, unsweetened or dietetic, solids & liq.:		
(Diet Delight) juice pack	½ cup	18.0
(Libby's) Lite	½ cup	16.0
(S&W) *Nutradiet*	1 slice	7.5
PINEAPPLE, CANDIED	1-oz. serving	22.7
PINEAPPLE & GRAPEFRUIT JUICE DRINK, canned:		

Food and Description	*Measure or Quantity*	*Carbohydrates (grams)*
(Del Monte) regular or pink	6 fl. oz.	24.0
(Dole) pink	6 fl. oz.	25.4
(Texsun)	6 fl. oz.	22.0
PINEAPPLE JUICE:		
Canned:		
(Del Monte)	6 fl. oz.	25.0
(Dole)	6 fl. oz.	25.4
(Texsun)	6 fl. oz.	24.0
*Frozen (Minute Maid)	6 fl. oz.	22.7
PINEAPPLE-ORANGE JUICE:		
Canned (Del Monte)	6 fl. oz.	24.0
*Frozen (Minute Maid)	6 fl. oz.	23.0
PINE NUT, pignolias, shelled	1 oz.	3.3
PINOT CHARDONNAY WINE		
(Paul Masson) 12% alcohol	3 fl. oz.	2.4
PISTACHIO NUT:		
In shell	½ cup	6.3
Shelled	¼ cup	5.9
(Fisher) shelled, roasted, salted	1 oz.	5.4
PIZZA PIE:		
Regular, non-frozen:		
Home recipe	⅛ of 14″ pie	21.2
(Pizza Hut):		
Cheese	½ of 10″ pie	53.2
Pepperoni	½ of 10″ pie	54.4
Frozen:		
Canadian style bacon (Celeste)	8-oz. pie	50.4
Cheese:		
(Celeste)	¼ of 19-oz. pie	31.6
(Stouffer's) French Bread	½ of 10¼-oz. pkg.	43.0
(Weight Watchers)	6-oz. pie	37.0
Combination:		
(Celeste) Chicago style	¼ of 24-oz. pie	36.2
(La Pizzeria)	½ of 13½-oz. pie	43.0
(Van de Kamp's) thick crust	¼ of 24½-oz. pie	24.0
(Weight Watchers)	7¼-oz. pie	38.0
Deluxe:		
(Celeste)	9-oz. pie	62.7
(Stouffer's) French Bread	½ of 12⅜-oz. pkg.	46.0
Hamburger (Stouffer's) French Bread	½ of 12 ¼-oz. pkg.	39.0
Mexican style (Van de Kamp's)	½ of 11-oz. pkg.	27.0
Pepperoni:		
(Stouffer's) French Bread	½ of 11½-oz. pkg.	44.0
(Van de Kamp's) thick crust	¼ of 22-oz. pie	38.0

Food and Description	*Measure or Quantity*	*Carbohydrates (grams)*
Sausage:		
(Celeste)	8-oz. pie	59.6
(Stouffer's) French Bread	½ of 12-oz. pkg.	44.0
(Weight Watchers) veal	6¾-oz. pie	35.1
Sausage & mushroom:		
(Celeste)	¼ of 24-oz. pie	34.1
(Stouffer's) French Bread	½ of 12½-oz. pkg.	40.0
Sicilian style (Celeste) deluxe	¼ of 26-oz. pie	45.4
Supreme (Celeste) without meat	8-oz. pie	49.2
Vegetable (Weight Watchers)	7 ¼-oz. pie	39.0
PIZZA SAUCE:		
(Contadina)	½ cup	10.0
(Ragu) regular or *Pizza Quick*	3 T.	6.0
PLUM:		
Fresh, Japanese & hybrid	2" plum	6.9
Fresh, prune-type, halves	½ cup	15.8
Canned, regular pack		
(Stokely-Van Camp)	½ cup	30.0
Canned, unsweetened, purple, solids & liq.:		
(Diet Delight) juice pack	½ cup	19.0
(Featherweight) water pack	½ cup	9.0
(S&W) *Nutradiet,* juice pack	½ cup	20.0
PLUM, PRESERVE OR JAM, sweetened (Smucker's)	1 T.	13.0
PLUM PUDDING		
(Richardson & Robbins)	2" wedge	61.0
POLYNESIAN-STYLE DINNER, frozen (Swanson) *TV Brand*	12-oz. dinner	46.0
POMEGRANATE, whole	1 lb.	41.7
PONDEROSA RESTAURANT:		
A-1 Sauce	1 tsp.	1.0
Beef, chopped (patty only)	Any type	0.
Beverages:		
Coca-Cola	8 fl. oz.	24.0
Coffee	6 fl. oz.	.5
Dr. Pepper	8 fl. oz.	24.8
Milk, chocolate	8 fl. oz.	25.9
Orange drink	8 fl. oz.	30.0
Root beer	8 fl. oz.	25.6
Sprite	8 fl. oz.	24.0
Tab	8 fl. oz.	.0
Bun:		
Regular	2.4-oz. bun	35.0
Hot dog	1 bun	18.9
Junior	1.4-oz. bun	21.0

Food and Description	*Measure or Quantity*	*Carbohydrates (grams)*
Steakhouse deluxe	2.4-oz. bun	35.0
Chicken strips:		
Adult portion	2¾ oz.	15.8
Child	1.4 oz.	7.9
Cocktail sauce	1½ oz.	14.5
Filet Mignon	3.8 oz. (edible portion).	.2
Filet of sole, fish only (See also Bun)	3-oz. piece	4.4
Fish, baked	4.9-oz. serving	11.6
Gelatin dessert	½ cup	23.5
Gravy, au jus	1 oz.	Tr.
Ham & cheese:		
Bun (See Bun)		
Cheese, Swiss	2 slices (.8 oz.)	.5
Ham	2½ oz.	1.4
Hot dog, child's, meat only (See also Bun)	1.6-oz. hot dog	2.0
Margarine:		
Pat	1 tsp.	Tr.
On potato, as served	½ oz.	.1
Mustard sauce, sweet & sour	1 oz.	9.5
New York strip steak	6.1 oz. (edible portion)	0.
Onion, chopped	1 T.	.9
Pickle, dill	3 slices (.7 oz.)	.2
Potato:		
Baked	7.2-oz. potato	32.8
French fries	3-oz. serving	30.2
Prime ribs	Any quantity	0.
Pudding, chocolate	4½ oz.	27.1
Ribeye	3.2 oz. (edible portion)	0.
Ribeye & Shrimp:		
Ribeye	3.2 oz.	0.
Shrimp	2.2 oz.	6.2
Roll, kaiser	2.2-oz. roll	33.0
Salad bar:		
Bean sprouts	1 oz.	1.5
Beets	1 oz.	.9
Broccoli	1 oz.	1.7
Cabbage, red	1 oz.	2.0
Carrots	1 oz.	2.8
Cauliflower	1 oz.	1.5
Celery	1 oz.	1.1
Chickpeas (Garbanzos)	1 oz.	17.3

Food and Description	*Measure or Quantity*	*Carbohydrates (grams)*
Cucumber	1 oz.	1.0
Mushrooms	1 oz.	1.2
Onion, white	1 oz.	2.6
Pepper, green	1 oz.	1.4
Radish	1 oz.	1.0
Tomato	1 oz.	1.3
Salad dressing:		
Blue cheese	1 oz.	2.1
Italian, creamy	1 oz.	2.8
Low calorie	1 oz.	.8
Oil & vinegar	1 oz.	.9
Thousand Island	1 oz.	9.2
Shrimp dinner	7 pieces (3½ oz.)	9.8
Sirloin	Any quantity	0.
Steak sauce	1 oz.	4.6
Tartar sauce	1.5 oz.	4.5
T-Bone	Any quantity	0.
Tomato (See also Salad Bar):		
Slices	2 slices (.9 oz.)	1.2
Whole, small	3.5 oz.	4.7
Topping, whipped	¼ oz.	1.2
Worcestershire sauce	1 tsp.	.9
POPCORN:		
*Plain, popped fresh:		
(Jiffy Pop) buttered	½ of 5-oz. pkg.	29.4
(Pillsbury) Microwave Popcorn:		
Regular	1 cup	6.0
Butter flavor	1 cup	6.5
Packaged:		
Plain (Bachman)	1 oz.	13.0
Caramel-coated:		
(Bachman)	1-oz. serving	25.0
(Old London) without peanuts	1 ¾-oz. serving	43.6
Cheese flavored (Bachman)	1-oz. serving	14.0
Cracker Jack	¾-oz. serving	16.7
***POPOVER MIX** (Flako)	1 popover	25.0
POPPY SEED (French's)	1 tsp.	.8
POPSICLE, twin pop	3-fl.-oz. pop	17.0
POP TARTS (See TOASTER CAKE OR PASTRY)		
PORK:	Any quantity	0.
PORK DINNER, frozen (Swanson)		
TV Brand	11 ¼-oz. dinner	20.0
PORK, PACKAGED (Eckrich)	1-oz. serving	1.0
PORK RINDS, *Baken-Ets*	1-oz. serving	1.0

Food and Description	*Measure or Quantity*	*Carbohydrates (grams)*
PORK STEAK, BREADED, FROZEN (Hormel)	3-oz. serving	11.0
PORT WINE:		
(Gallo)	3 fl. oz.	7.8
(Louis M. Martini)	3 fl. oz.	2.0
***POSTUM,** instant*	6 fl. oz.	2.0
POTATO:		
Cooked:		
Au gratin	½ cup	17.9
Baked, peeled	2½" dia. potato	20.9
Boiled, peeled	4.2-oz. potato	17.7
French-fried	10 pieces	20.5
Hash-browned, home recipe	½ cup	28.4
Mashed, milk & butter added	½ cup	12.1
Canned, solids & liq.:		
(Del Monte)	½ cup	10.0
(Sunshine) whole	½ cup	10.5
Frozen:		
(Birds Eye):		
Cottage fries	2.8-oz. serving	17.3
Crinkle cuts, regular	3-oz. serving	18.4
Farm style wedge	3-oz. serving	17.9
French fries, regular	3-oz. serving	16.8
Hash browns, shredded	¼ of 12-oz. pkg.	13.1
Tasti Puffs	¼ of 10-oz. pkg.	19.4
Tiny Taters	⅕ of 16-oz. pkg.	22.0
Whole peeled	3.2-oz.	12.8
(Green Giant):		
Sliced, in butter sauce	½ cup	14.0
& sweet peas in bacon cream sauce	½ cup	15.0
(McKenzie) whole, white	3.2 oz.	13.0
(Stouffer's):		
Au gratin	⅓ of pkg.	13.0
Scalloped	⅓ of pkg.	14.0
POTATO & BACON, canned (Hormel) *Short Orders,* au gratin	7½-oz. can	20.0
POTATO & BEEF, canned, *Dinty Moore* (Hormel) *Short Orders*	7½-oz. can	25.0
POTATO CHIP:		
(Bachman) any flavor	1 oz.	14.0
(Featherweight) unsalted	1 oz.	14.0
(Frito-Lay's) natural	1 oz.	14.1
Lay's, sour cream & onion flavor	1 oz.	15.0
Pringle's:		
Regular	1 oz.	10.8

Food and Description	*Measure or Quantity*	*Carbohydrates (grams)*
Light	1 oz.	16.5
POTATO & HAM, canned (Hormel)		
Short Orders, scalloped	7½-oz. can	19.0
***POTATO MIX:**		
Au gratin:		
(Betty Crocker)	½ cup	21.0
(French's) *Big Tate,* tangy	½ cup	25.0
(Libby's) *Potato Classics*	¾ cup	22.0
Creamed (Betty Crocker) saucepan	½ cup	21.0
Hash browns (Betty Crocker) with onion	½ cup	23.0
Hickory smoke cheese (Betty Crocker)	½ cup	21.0
Julienne (Betty Crocker) with mild cheese sauce	½ cup	17.0
Mashed:		
(American Beauty)	½ cup	17.0
(Pillsbury) *Hungry Jack,* flakes	½ cup	17.0
Scalloped:		
(Betty Crocker)	½ cup	19.0
(French's) *Big Tate*	½ cup	25.0
(Libby's) *Potato Classics*	¾ cup	24.0
Sour cream & chive (Betty Crocker)	½ cup	19.0
***POTATO PANCAKE MIX**		
(French's) *Big Tate*	3" pancake	5.7
POTATO SALAD:		
Home recipe	½ cup	16.8
Canned (Nalley's) German style	4-oz. serving	18.2
POTATO STICKS (Durkee) *O & C*	1½-oz. can	22.0
POTATO, STUFFED, BAKED, frozen (Green Giant):		
With cheese flavored topping	½ of 10-oz. pkg.	33.0
With sour cream & chives	½ of 10-oz. pkg.	31.0
POTATO TOPPERS (Libby's)	1 T.	4.0
POUND CAKE (See CAKE, Pound)		
PRESERVE OR JAM (See individual flavors)		
PRETZEL:		
(Bachman) regular or butter	1 oz.	21.0
(Featherweight) unsalted	1 piece	1.3
(Nabisco) *Mister Salty,* Dutch	1 piece	11.0
PRODUCT 19, cereal (Kellogg's)	1 cup	24.0
PROSCIUTTO (Hormel)	1 oz.	0.
PRUNE:		
Canned:		
(Featherweight) stewed,		

Food and Description	*Measure or Quantity*	*Carbohydrates (grams)*
water pack	½ cup	35.0
(Sunsweet) stewed	½ cup	32.0
Dried:		
(Del Monte)	2 oz.	30.0
(Sunsweet) whole	2 oz.	32.0
PRUNE JUICE:		
(Del Monte)	6 fl. oz.	33.0
(Mott's) regular	6 fl. oz.	34.0
(Sunsweet) with pulp	6 fl. oz.	32.0
PRUNE NECTAR, canned (Mott's)	6 fl. oz.	24.0
PUDDING OR PIE FILLING:		
Canned, regular pack:		
Banana:		
(Del Monte) *Pudding Cup*	5-oz. container	30.1
(Hunt's) *Snack Pack*	5-oz. container	24.0
Butterscotch:		
(Del Monte) *Pudding Cup*	5-oz. container	30.8
(Hunt's) *Snack Pack*	5-oz. container	27.0
Chocolate:		
(Del Monte) *Pudding Cup*	5-oz. container	32.9
(Hunt's) *Snack Pack*	5-oz. container	28.0
Rice (Comstock; Menner's)	½ of 7½-oz. can	23.0
Tapioca:		
(Del Monte) *Pudding Cup*	5-oz. container	30.1
(Hunt's) *Snack Pack*	5-oz. container	23.0
Vanilla (Del Monte)	5-oz. container	32.1
Canned, dietetic pack (Sego) all flavors	4-oz. serving	39.0
Chilled, *Swiss Miss:*		
Butterscotch or chocolate malt	4-oz. container	22.0
Chocolate	4-oz. container	25.0
Vanilla	4-oz. container	24.0
Frozen (Rich's):		
Banana	3-oz. container	19.3
Butterscotch or vanilla	4½-oz. container	27.4
Chocolate	4½-oz. container	27.1
*Mix, sweetened, regular & instant:		
Banana:		
(Jell-O) cream, regular	½ cup	26.7
(Royal) regular	½ cup	27.0
Butter pecan (Jell-O) instant	½ cup	29.1
Butterscotch:		
(Jell-O) instant	½ cup	30.0
(My-T-Fine) regular	½ cup	28.0
Chocolate:		
(Jell-O) regular	½ cup	28.8

Food and Description	*Measure or Quantity*	*Carbohydrates (grams)*
(My-T-Fine) regular	½ cup	27.8
Coconut:		
(Jell-O) cream, regular	½ cup	24.4
(Royal) instant	½ cup	30.0
Custard (Royal) regular	½ cup	22.0
Flan (Royal) regular	½ cup	22.0
Lemon:		
(Jell-O) instant	½ cup	31.1
(My-T-Fine) regular	½ cup	30.0
Lime (Royal) Key Lime, regular	½ cup	30.0
Pineapple (Jell-O) cream, regular	½ cup	30.4
Pistachio (Royal) nut, instant	½ cup	30.0
Raspberry (Salada) *Danish Dessert*	½ cup	32.0
Rice, *Jell-O Americana*	½ cup	29.9
Strawberry (Salada) *Danish Dessert*	½ cup	32.0
Tapioca:		
Jell-O Americana, chocolate	½ cup	27.8
(My-T-Fine) vanilla	½ cup	28.0
Vanilla:		
(Jell-O) French, regular	½ cup	29.7
(Royal)	½ cup	29.0
*Mix, dietetic:		
Butterscotch:		
(Dia-Mel)	½ cup	9.0
(D-Zerta)	½ cup	12.0
Chocolate:		
(Dia-Mel; Louis Sherry)	½ cup	9.0
(D-Zerta)	½ cup	11.5
(Estee)	½ cup	12.0
Lemon:		
(Dia-Mel)	½ cup	4.0
(Estee)	½ cup	12.0
Vanilla:		
(Dia-Mel)	½ cup	9.0
(Estee)	½ cup	13.0
(Featherweight) artificially sweetened	½ cup	9.0
PUFFED RICE:		
(Malt-O-Meal)	1 cup	12.0
(Quaker)	1 cup	12.7
PUFFED WHEAT:		
(Malt-O-Meal)	1 cup	11.0

Food and Description	*Measure or Quantity*	*Carbohydrates (grams)*
(Quaker)	1 cup	10.0
PUMPKIN, canned (Libby's) solid pack	½ cup	20.0
PUMPKIN SEED, in hull	1 oz.	3.2

Q

Food and Description	*Measure or Quantity*	*Carbohydrates (grams)*
QUIK (Nestlé) chocolate	1 tsp.	9.5
QUISP, cereal	1 ⅙ cup	23.1

R

Food and Description	Measure or Quantity	Carbohydrates (grams)
RADISH	2 small radishes	.7
RAISIN, dried:		
(Del Monte)	3 oz.	68.0
(Sun-Maid) Thompson, seedless	1 oz.	23.0
RAISINS, RICE & RYE, cereal		
(Kellogg's)	¾ cup	31.0
RALSTON, cereal	¼ cup	20.0
RASPBERRY:		
Fresh:		
Black, trimmed	½ cup	10.5
Red, trimmed	½ cup	9.8
Frozen (Birds Eye) quick thaw	5-oz. serving	37.0
RASPBERRY PRESERVE OR JAM:		
Sweetened (Smucker's)	1 T.	13.5
Dietetic:		
(Dia-Mel; Louis Sherry)	1 T.	0.
(Featherweight) red	1 T.	4.0
(S&W) *Nutradiet,* red	1 T.	3.0
RATOTOUILLE, frozen (Stouffer's)	5-oz. serving	9.0
RAVIOLI:		
Canned, regular pack (Franco-American):		
Beef, *RavioliOs*	7½-oz. serving	34.0
Cheese, in tomato sauce, *RavioliOs*	7½-oz. serving	39.0
Canned, dietetic (Dia-Mel) beef	8-oz. can	35.0
RELISH:		
Hamburger (Nalley's)	1 T.	4.1
Hot dog (Nalley's)	1 T.	4.8
Sweet (Smucker's)	1 T.	3.3
RENNET MIX (Junket):		
*Powder, any flavor:		
Made with skim milk	½ cup	15.0

Food and Description	*Measure or Quantity*	*Carbohydrates (grams)*
Made with whole milk	½ cup	16.0
Tablet	1 tablet	0.
RHINE WINE:		
(Great Western)	3 fl. oz.	2.9
(Taylor)	3 fl. oz.	3.0
RHUBARB, cooked, sweetened	½ cup	43.2
***RICE:**		
Brown (Uncle Ben's) parboiled	⅔ cup	26.4
White:		
(Minute Rice) instant	⅔ cup	27.4
(Success) long grain	½ cup	20.0
White & wild (Carolina)	½ cup	20.0
RICE, FRIED (See also RICE MIX):		
*Canned, (La Choy)	⅓ of 11-oz. can	40.0
Frozen:		
(Birds Eye)	3.7-oz. serving	22.8
(Green Giant) shrimp	10-oz. entree	49.0
(La Choy) & pork	8-oz. serving	52.0
***RICE, FRIED, SEASONING MIX**		
(Kikkoman)	1-oz. pkg.	15.6
RICE KRINKLES, cereal (Post)	⅞ cup	25.9
RICE KRISPIES, cereal (Kellogg's)	1 cup	25.0
RICE MIX:		
Beef:		
*(Carolina) *Bake-It-Easy*	¼ of pkg.	23.0
(Minute Rice)	½ cup	25.0
Rice-A-Roni	⅙ of 8-oz. pkg.	26.0
Chicken:		
*(Carolina) *Bake-It-Easy*	¼ of pkg.	23.0
Rice-A-Roni	⅕ of 8-oz. pkg.	33.2
*Fried (Minute Rice)	½ cup	25.2
Long grain & wild (Minute Rice)	½ cup	25.0
*Oriental (Carolina) *Bake-It-Easy*	½ of pkg.	23.0
Spanish:		
*(Carolina) *Bake-It-Easy*	¼ of pkg.	23.0
*(Minute Rice)	½ cup	25.6
Rice-A-Roni	⅙ of 7½-oz. pkg.	25.9
RICE, SPANISH, canned:		
Regular pack (Comstock; Menner's)	½ of 7½-oz. can	27.0
Dietetic (Featherweight) low sodium	7½-oz. serving	30.0
Frozen (Birds Eye)	3.7-oz. serving	26.1
RICE & VEGETABLE, frozen:		
(Birds Eye):		
French style	3.7-oz. serving	25.0
Peas with mushrooms	2⅓ oz.	23.1

Food and Description	Measure or Quantity	Carbohydrates (grams)
(Green Giant) *Rice Originals*		
& broccoli in cheese sauce or festive	½ cup	19.0
& herb butter sauce	½ cup	21.0
Pilaf	½ cup	23.0
RICE WINE:		
Chinese, 20.7% alcohol	1 fl. oz.	1.1
Japanese, 10.6% alcohol	1 fl. oz.	13.1
ROCK & RYE (Mr. Boston)	1 fl. oz.	7.2
ROE, baked or broiled, cod & shad	4 oz.	2.2
ROLL OR BUN:		
Commercial type, non-frozen:		
Biscuit (Wonder)	1-oz. piece	14.0
Brown & serve (Wonder)		
Gem Style	1-oz. piece	13.0
Crescent (Pepperidge Farm)		
butter	1-oz. piece	14.0
Croissant (Pepperidge Farm):		
Butter	2-oz. piece	19.0
Chocolate	2.4-oz. piece	25.0
Walnut	2-oz. piece	21.0
Dinner:		
Home Pride	1-oz. piece	14.0
(Pepperidge Farm)	.7-oz. piece	10.0
Finger (Pepperidge Farm) sesame or poppy seed	.6-oz. piece	9.0
Frankfurter:		
(Arnold) hot dog	1.3-oz. piece	20.0
(Pepperidge Farm)	1¾-oz. piece	18.0
(Wonder)	1-oz. piece	14.0
French:		
(Arnold) *Francisco*, sourdough	1.1-oz. piece	16.0
(Pepperidge Farm):		
Small	1.3-oz. piece	20.0
Large	3-oz. piece	44.0
Hamburger:		
(Arnold)	1.4-oz. piece	21.0
(Pepperidge Farm)	1.5-oz. piece	23.0
Roman Meal	1.8-oz. piece	36.1
Hoggie (Wonder)	5-oz. piece	73.0
Honey (Hostess) glazed	3.75-oz. piece	49.0
Old fashioned (Pepperidge Farm)	.6-oz. piece	23.0
Pan (Wonder)	1-oz. piece	14.0
Parkerhouse (Pepperidge Farm)	.6-oz. piece	9.0
Party (Pepperidge Farm)	.4-oz. piece	22.0
Sandwich (Arnold) soft	1.3-oz. piece	18.0

Food and Description	*Measure or Quantity*	*Carbohydrates (grams)*
Soft (Pepperidge Farm)	1 ¼-oz. piece	18.0
Frozen:		
Apple crunch (Sara Lee)	1-oz. piece	13.5
Caramel pecan (Sara Lee)	1.3-oz. piece	17.4
Cinnamon (Sara Lee)	.9-oz. piece	13.9
Croissant (Sara Lee)	.9-oz. piece	11.2
Crumb (Sara Lee) French	1 ¾-oz. piece	29.9
Danish (Sara Lee):		
Apple	1.3-oz. piece	17.4
Cheese	1.3-oz. piece	13.9
Cinnamon raisin	1.3-oz. piece	17.3
Pecan	1.3-oz. piece	18.3
Honey (Morton) mini	1.3-oz. piece	18.0
***ROLL OR BUN DOUGH:**		
Frozen (Rich's):		
Cinnamon	2¼-oz. piece	32.8
Franfurter	1 piece	24.9
Hamburger, regular	1 piece	25.0
Parkerhouse	1 piece	13.4
Refrigerated (Pillsbury):		
Caramel danish, with nuts	1 piece	19.5
Cinnamon raisin danish	1 piece	19.5
Crescent	1 piece	11.0
White, bakery style	1 piece	20.0
***ROLL MIX, HOT** (Pillsbury)	1 piece	17.0
ROMAN MEAL CEREAL, 2 or 5 minute	⅓ cup	20.0
ROSE WINE:		
(Great Western)	3 fl. oz.	2.4
(Paul Masson):		
Regular, 11.8% alcohol	3 fl. oz.	4.2
Light, 7.1% alcohol	3 fl. oz.	3.9
RUTABAGA:		
Canned (Sunshine) solids & liq.	½ cup	6.9
Frozen (Southland)	4 oz.	13.0

S

Food and Description	Measure or Quantity	Carbohydrates (grams)
SAFFLOWER SEED, in hull	1 oz.	1.9
SAGE (French's)	1 tsp.	.6
SAKE WINE	1 fl. oz.	1.4
SALAD CRUNCHIES (Libby's)	1 T.	4.0
SALAD DRESSING:		
Regular:		
Bacon (Seven Seas) creamy	1 T.	1.0
Bleu or blue cheese:		
(Bernstein) Danish	1 T.	.6
(Wish-Bone) chunky	1 T.	1.0
Caesar:		
(Pfeiffer)	1 T.	1.0
(Seven Seas) *Viva*	1 T.	1.0
Cheddar & bacon (Wish-Bone)	1 T.	1.0
Cucumber (Wish-Bone)	1 T.	2.0
French:		
(Bernstein's) creamy	1 T.	2.1
(Seven Seas) creamy	1 T.	2.0
(Wish-Bone) deluxe or garlic	1 T.	2.0
Garlic (Wish-Bone) creamy	1 T.	2.0
Green Goddess (Seven Seas)	1 T.	0.
Herb & spice (Seven Seas)	1 T.	1.0
Italian:		
(Seven Seas)	1 T.	1.0
(Wish-Bone) creamy	1 T.	2.0
Red wine & vinegar & oil (Seven Seas)	1 T.	1.0
Roquefort:		
(Bernstein's)	1 T.	.8
(Marie's)	1 T.	1.1
Russian:		
(Pfeiffer)	1 T.	4.0
(Wish-Bone)	1 T.	7.0
Thousand Island:		

Food and Description	*Measure or Quantity*	*Carbohydrates (grams)*
(Pfeiffer)	1 T.	2.0
(Wish-Bone) regular	1 T.	2.0
Vinaigrette (Bernstein's) French	1 T.	.2
Dietetic or low calorie:		
Bleu or blue cheese:		
(Dia-Mel)	1 T.	Tr.
(Tillie Lewis) *Tasti-Diet*	1 T.	Tr.
(Walden Farms) chunky	1 T.	1.7
(Wish-Bone)	1 T.	3.0
Caesar:		
(Estee) garlic	1 T.	1.0
(Featherweight) creamy	1 T.	2.0
Cucumber (Dia-Mel) creamy	1 T.	Tr.
Cucumber & onion (Featherweight) creamy	1 T.	0.
French:		
(Walden Farms) chunky	1 T.	2.6
(Wish-Bone) regular	1 T.	2.0
Garlic (Dia-Mel)	1 T.	0.
Italian:		
(Estee) spicy	1 T.	1.0
(Tillie Lewis) *Tasti Diet*	1 T.	0.
(Weight Watchers)	1 T.	2.0
(Wish-Bone)	1 T.	1.0
Onion & chive (Wish-Bone)	1 T.	3.0
Red wine/vinegar (Featherweight)	1 T.	1.06
Russian:		
(Featherweight) creamy	1 T.	1.0
(Weight Watchers)	1 T.	2.0
(Wish-Bone)	1 T.	5.0
Tahiti (Dia-Mel)	1 T.	Tr.
Thousand Island:		
(Walden Farms)	1 T.	3.1
(Weight Watchers)	1 T.	2.0
(Wish-Bone)	1 T.	3.0
2-Calorie Low Sodium (Featherweight)	1 T.	0.
Whipped (Tillie Lewis) *Tasti Diet*	1 T.	1.0
Yogurt buttermilk (Diet-Mel)	1 T.	Tr.
SALAD DRESSING MIX:		
*Regular (Good Seasons):		
Blue cheese	1 T.	.3
French, old fashioned	1 T.	.5
Garlic, cheese	1 T.	.5
Italian, regular or cheese	1 T.	.6
Tomato & herbs	1 T.	1.0

Food and Description	*Measure or Quantity*	*Carbohydrates (grams)*
Dietetic:		
*Blue cheese (Weight Watchers)	1 T.	1.0
*French (Weight Watchers)	1 T.	1.0
*Italian:		
(Good Seasons) regular	1 T.	1.8
(Weight Watchers):		
Regular	1 T.	0.
Creamy	1 T.	1.0
*Russian (Weight Watchers)	1 T.	1.0
*Thousand Island (Weight Watchers)	1 T.	1.0
SALAMI:		
(Eckrich) hard	1-oz. serving	1.0
(Hormel):		
Beef or Genoa	1-oz. serving	0.
Hard	1-oz. serving	0.
(Oscar Mayer):		
For beer, beef	.8-oz. serving	.2
Cotto	.8-oz. slice	.4
SALISBURY STEAK, frozen:		
(Banquet):		
Buffet Supper	2-lb. pkg.	30.0
Extra Helping	19-oz. dinner	72.0
(Green Giant) with gravy, oven bake	7-oz. serving	11.0
(Morton) *Country Table*	15-oz. dinner	62.0
(Stouffer's) *Lean Cuisine*	9½-oz. pkg.	14.0
(Swanson):		
Regular, with gravy	10-oz. entree	14.0
TV Brand	11½-oz. dinner	43.0
SALMON, FRESH OR CANNED	Any quantity	0.
SALMON, SMOKED (Vita):		
Lox, drained	4-oz. jar	.2
Nova, drained	4-oz. can	1.0
SALT:		
Table (Morton)	Any quantity	0.
Substitute:		
(Adolph's) plain	1 tsp.	Tr.
Salt-It (Dia-Mel)	1 tsp.	0.
SANDWICH SPREAD:		
(Hellman's)	1 T.	2.2
(Oscar Mayer)	1-oz. serving	3.2
SANGRIA (Taylor)	3 fl. oz.	10.8
SARDINE, canned:		
Atlantic (Del Monte) with tomato sauce	7½-oz. can	3.8

Food and Description	*Measure or Quantity*	*Carbohydrates (grams)*
Imported (Underwood) in mustard or tomato sauce	3¾-oz. can	1.0
Norwegian, *King Oscar Brand:*		
In mustard or tomato sauce	3 ¾-oz. can	2.0
In oil, drained	3-oz. can	1.0
SAUCE:		
Regular:		
A-1	1 T.	3.1
Barbecue:		
Chris & Pitt's	1 T.	4.0
(Gold's)	1 T.	3.9
Open Pit (General Foods) original, hot n' spicy or smoke flavor	1 T.	5.5
Burrito (Del Monte)	¼ cup	4.0
Chili (See CHILI SAUCE)		
Cocktail:		
(Gold's)	1 T.	7.5
(Pfeiffer)	1-oz. serving	12.0
Escoffier Sauce Diable	1 T.	4.3
Escoffier Sauce Robert	1 T.	5.1
Famous Sauce	1 T.	2.2
Hot, *Frank's*	1 tsp.	0.
Italian (See also SPAGHETTI SAUCE or TOMATO SAUCE):		
(Contadina)	4-oz. serving	10.5
(Ragu) red coking	3½-oz. serving	6.0
Salsa Mexicana (Contadina)	4 fl. oz.	6.8
Salsa Picante (Del Monte)	¼ cup	4.0
Salsa Roja (Del Monte)	¼ cup	4.0
Seafood cocktail (Del Monte)	1 T.	4.9
Soy:		
(Gold's)	1 T.	1.0
(Kikkoman) regular	1 T.	.9
(La Choy)	1 T.	.9
Spare rib (Gold's)	1 T.	3.9
Steak Supreme	1 T.	5.1
Sweet & sour:		
(Contadina)	4 fl. oz.	29.6
(La Choy)	1-oz. serving	12.6
Tabasco	¼ tsp.	Tr.
Taco:		
Old El Paso	1-oz. serving	2.3
(Ortega)	1 T.	5.1

Food and Description	*Measure or Quantity*	*Carbohydrates (grams)*
Tartar:		
(Hellman's)	1 T.	.2
(Nalley's)	1 T.	.3
Teriyaki (Kikkoman)	1 T.	3.1
V-8	1-oz. serving	6.0
White, medium	¼ cup	6.4
Worcestershire:		
(French's) regular or smoky	1 T.	2.0
(Gold's)	1 T.	3.3
Dietetic (Estee):		
Barbecue	1 T.	4.0
Cocktail	1 T.	3.0
SAUCE MIX:		
Regular:		
A la King (Durkee)	1-oz. pkg.	14.0
*Cheese:		
(Durkee)	½ cup	9.5
(French's)	½ cup	14.0
Hollandaise:		
(Durkee)	1-oz. pkg.	11.0
*(French's)	1 T.	.7
*Sour cream (French's)	2½ T.	5.0
*Sweet & sour (Durkee)	1 cup	45.0
Teriyaki (Kikkoman)	1.5-oz. pkg.	22.3
*White (Durkee)	1 cup	41.0
*Dietetic (Weight Watchers) lemon butter	1 T.	1.0
SAUERKRAUT, canned:		
(Claussen) drained	½ cup	2.8
(Del Monte) solids & liq.	½ cup	6.0
(Silver Floss) solids & liq.:		
Regular	½ cup	5.0
Krispy Kraut	½ cup	5.0
SAUSAGE:		
*Brown & serve (Swift) original	.8-oz. link	.5
Polish-style (Eckrich) beer	1-oz. serving	1.0
Pork:		
*(Hormel) *Little Sizzlers*	1 link	0.
(Jimmy Dean)	2-oz. serving	Tr.
*(Oscar Mayer) *Little Friers*	1-oz. link	.2
Roll (Eckrich)	1-oz. slice	1.0
Smoked:		
(Eckrich) beef, *Smok-Y-Links*	.8-oz. link	1.0
(Hormel) smokies	1 sausage	.5
(Oscar Mayer) beef	1½-oz. link	.9
*Turkey (Louis Rich) links or tube	1-oz. serving	Tr.

Food and Description	*Measure or Quantity*	*Carbohydrates (grams)*
Vienna (Libby's) in beef broth	1 link	.3
SAUTERNE:		
(Great Western)	3 fl. oz.	4.5
(Taylor)	3 fl. oz.	4.8
SCALLOP:		
Raw	4-oz. serving	3.7
Frozen (Mrs. Paul's) breaded & fried	3½-oz. serving	23.0
SCHNAPPS, APPLE (Mr. Boston)	1 fl. oz.	8.0
SCHNAPPS, PEPPERMINT (Mr. Boston)	1 fl. oz.	8.0
SCREWDRIVER COCKTAIL (Mr. Boston) 12½% alcohol	3 fl. oz.	12.0
SEAFOOD PLATTER, frozen (Mrs. Paul's) breaded & fried	9-oz. serving	49.0
***SEGO* DIET FOOD,** canned:		
Chocolate or coconut	10-fl.-oz. can	39.0
Very banana or very butterscotch	10-fl.-oz. can	34.0
SELTZER (Canada Dry)	Any quantity	0.
SERUTAN	1 tsp.	1.3
SESAME SEEDS (French's)	1 tsp.	.9
SHAD, CREOLE	4-oz. serving	1.8
SHAKE'N BAKE:		
Chicken, original	1 pkg.	41.6
Crispy country milk	1 pkg.	40.4
Fish	2-oz. pkg.	17.0
Italian	1 pkg.	41. 2
Pork, barbecue	1 pkg.	59.2
SHELLS, PASTA, STUFFED, frozen (Stouffer's) cheese stuffed	9-oz. serving	26.0
SHERBET:		
(Baskin-Robbins) Daiquiri Ice or orange	1 scoop	20.9
(Howard Johnson's)	½ cup	29.0
(Meadow Gold) orange	¼ pint	26.0
SHERRY:		
Cream (Great Western) Solera	3 fl. oz.	12.2
Dry (Williams & Humbert)	3 fl. oz.	4.5
Dry Sack (Williams & Humbert)	3 fl. oz.	4.5
SHREDDED WHEAT:		
(Nabisco):		
Regular size	¾-oz. biscuit	19.0
Spoon Size	⅔ cup	23.0
(Quaker)	1 biscuit	11.0
SHRIMP:		
Raw, meat only	4 oz.	1.7

Food and Description	*Measure or Quantity*	*Carbohydrates (grams)*
Canned (Bumble Bee) solids & liq.	4½-oz. can	.9
Frozen (Mrs. Paul's)		
breaded & fried	3-oz. serving	15.0
SHRIMP DINNER, frozen:		
(Stouffer's) Newburg	6½-oz. serving	4.0
(Van de Kamp's)	10-oz. dinner	40.0
SLENDER **(Carnation):**		
Bar	1 bar	13.0
Dry	1 packet	21.0
Liquid	10-fl.-oz. can	34.0
SLOPPY HOT DOG SEASONING MIX (French's)	1½-oz. pkg.	28.0
SLOPPY JOE:		
Canned:		
(Hormel) *Short Orders*	7½-oz. can	15.0
(Libby's):		
Beef	⅓ cup	7.0
Pork	⅓ cup	6.0
Frozen (Banquet) *Cookin' Bag*	5-oz. pkg.	12.0
SLOPPY JOE SEASONING MIX:		
*(Durkee) pizza flavor	1¼ cups	26.0
(French's)	1½-oz. pkg.	32.0
(McCormick)	1.3-oz. pkg.	23.4
***SMURF BERRY CRUNCH*, cereal** (Post)	1 cup	25.4
SNACK BAR (Pepperidge Farm):		
Apple nut	1.7-oz. piece	33.0
Blueberry or brownie nut	1.7-oz. piece	36.0
Chocolate chip or coconut macaroon	1½-oz. piece	28.0
SNO BALL (Hostess)	1 piece	27.3
SOAVE WINE (Antinori)	3 fl. oz.	6.3
SOFT DRINK		
Sweetened:		
Birch beer (Canada Dry)	6 fl. oz.	21.0
Bitter lemon:		
(Canada Dry)	6 fl. oz.	19.5
(Schweppes)	6 fl. oz.	20.8
Bubble Up	6 fl. oz.	18.4
Cactus Cooler (Canada Dry)	6 fl. oz.	21.8
Cherry:		
(Canada Dry) wild	6 fl. oz.	24.0
(Shasta) black	6 fl. oz.	21.5
Chocolate (Yoo-Hoo)	6 fl. oz.	18.0
Club	Any quantity	0.
Cola:		
Coca-Cola:		

Food and Description	*Measure or Quantity*	*Carbohydrates (grams)*
Regular	6 fl. oz.	19.0
Caffeine-free	6 fl. oz.	20.0
Pepsi-Cola, regular or *Pepsi Free*	6 fl. oz.	19.8
(Shasta) regular	6 fl. oz.	19.5
Collins mix (Canada Dry)	6 fl. oz.	15.0
Cream:		
(Canada Dry) vanilla	6 fl. oz.	24.0
(Schweppes) red	6 fl. oz.	21.3
(Shasta)	6 fl. oz.	20.5
Dr. Pepper	6 fl. oz.	19.4
Fruit punch:		
(Nehi)	6 fl. oz.	22.8
(Shasta)	6 fl. oz.	23.0
Ginger ale:		
(Canada Dry) regular	6 fl. oz.	15.8
(Fanta)	6 fl. oz.	16.0
(Shasta)	6 fl. oz.	16.0
Ginger beer (Schweppes)	6 fl. oz.	16.8
Grape:		
(Canada Dry) concord	6 fl. oz.	24.0
(Fanta; Nehi)	6 fl. oz.	22.0
(Hi-C)	6 fl. oz.	20.0
(Schweppes)	6 fl. oz.	23.8
(Welch's) sparkling	6 fl. oz.	23.0
Half & half (Canada Dry)	6 fl. oz.	19.5
Hi-Spot (Canada Dry)	6 fl. oz.	18.7
Lemon (Hi-C)	6 fl. oz.	18.0
Mello Yello	6 fl. oz.	22.0
Mountain Dew	6 fl. oz.	22.2
Mr. PiBB	6 fl. oz.	19.0
Orange:		
(Canada Dry) *Sunrise*	6 fl. oz.	24.7
(Hi-C)	6 fl. oz.	20.0
(Sunkist)	6 fl. oz.	24.0
Peach (Nehi)	6 fl. oz.	23.0
Pineapple (Canada Dry)	6 fl. oz.	19.5
Quinine or tonic water (Canada Dry; Schweppes)	6 fl. oz.	16.5
Root beer:		
Barrelhead (Canada Dry)	6 fl. oz.	19.5
(Dad's)	6 fl. oz.	20.7
Rooti (Canada Dry)	6 fl. oz.	19.5
(Shasta) draft	6 fl. oz.	20.5
Seven-Up	6 fl. oz.	18.1
Sprite	6 fl. oz.	18.0

Food and Description	*Measure or Quantity*	*Carbohydrates (grams)*
Strawberry (Shasta)	6 fl. oz.	19.5
Tahitian Treat (Canada Dry)	6 fl. oz.	24.0
Upper Ten (Royal Crown)	6 fl. oz.	19.0
Wink (Canada Dry)	6 fl. oz.	22.5
Dietetic:		
Bubble Up	6 fl. oz.	Tr.
Cherry (Shasta) black	6 fl. oz.	Tr.
Chocolate (No-Cal)	6 fl. oz.	Tr.
Coffee (No-Cal)	6 fl. oz.	Tr.
Cola:		
(Canada Dry; No-Cal)	6 fl. oz.	0.
Coca Cola, regular or caffeine free	6 fl. oz.	.1
Diet Rite	6 fl. oz.	.1
Pepsi, diet, or caffeine free	6 fl. oz.	.1
Cream (Shasta)	6 fl. oz.	Tr.
Dr. Pepper	6 fl. oz.	.4
Fresca	6 fl. oz.	Tr.
Ginger Ale:		
(Canada Dry)	6 fl. oz.	0.
(No-Cal)	6 fl. oz.	0.
Grape (Shasta)	6 fl. oz.	Tr.
Grapefruit (Shasta)	6 fl. oz.	.2
Mr. PiBB	6 fl. oz.	.2
Orange:		
(Canada Dry; No-Cal)	6 fl. oz.	Tr.
(Shasta)	6 fl. oz.	Tr.
Quinine or tonic (No-Cal)	6 fl. oz.	Tr.
RC 100 (Royal Crown) caffeine free	6 fl. oz.	.1
Root beer:		
Barrelhead (Canada Dry)	6 fl. oz.	0.
(Dad's; Ramblin'; Shasta)	6 fl. oz.	.2
Seven-Up	6 fl. oz.	0.
Sprite	6 fl. oz.	Tr.
Tab, regular or caffeine free	6 fl. oz.	.2
SOLE, frozen:		
(Mrs. Paul's) fillets, breaded & fried	6-oz. serving	19.0
(Van de Kamp's) batter dipped, french fried	1 piece	12.0
(Weight Watchers) in lemon sauce	9⅛-oz. meal	17.0
SOUFFLE, frozen (Stouffer's cheese)	6-oz. serving	14.0
SOUP:		
Canned, regular pack:		

Food and Description	*Measure or Quantity*	*Carbohydrates (grams)*
*Asparagus (Campbell), condensed, cream of	8-oz. serving	11.0
Bean:		
(Campbell):		
Chunky, with ham, old fashioned	11-oz. can	37.0
*Condensed, with bacon	8-oz. serving	21.0
(Grandma Brown's)	8-oz. serving	29.1
Bean, black:		
*(Campbell) condensed	8-oz. serving	17.0
(Crosse & Blackwell)	6½-oz. serving	18.0
Beef:		
(Campbell):		
Chunky:		
Regular	10¾-oz. can	23.0
With noodles	10¾-oz. can	28.0
*Condensed:		
Regular	8-oz. serving	10.0
Broth, & noodles	8-oz. serving	9.0
Consomme	8-oz. serving	2.0
Noodle	8-oz. serving	7.0
Teriyaki	8-oz. serving	9.0
(College Inn) broth	1 cup	1.0
(Swanson)	7½-oz. can	1.0
Celery:		
*(Campbell) condensed, cream of	8-oz. serving	8.0
*(Rokeach):		
Prepared with milk	10-oz. serving	19.0
Prepared with water	10-oz. serving	12.0
*Cheddar cheese (Campbell)	8-oz. serving	10.0
Chicken:		
(Campbell):		
Chunky:		
Regular	10¾-oz. can	20.0
& rice	19-oz. can	30.0
Vegetable	19-oz. can	38.0
*Condensed:		
Alphabet	8-oz. serving	10.0
Broth:		
Plain	8-oz. serving	3.0
& rice	8-oz. serving	8.0
Cream of	8-oz. serving	9.0
Mushroom, creamy	8-oz. serving	9.0
NoodleOs	8-oz. serving	8.0
& rice	8-oz. serving	7.0

Food and Description	*Measure or Quantity*	*Carbohydrates (grams)*
Vegetable	8-oz. serving	8.0
*Semi-condensed, *Soup For One*, vegetable, full flavored	11-oz. serving	13.0
(College Inn) broth	1 cup	0.
(Swanson) broth	7¼-oz. can	3.0
Chili beef (Campbell) ***Chunky***	11-oz. can	37.0
Chowder:		
Beef'n vegetable (Hormel)	7½-oz. can	15.0
Chicken'n corn (Hormel)	7½-oz. can	15.0
Clam:		
Manhattan style:		
(Campbell):		
Chunky	19-oz. can	44.0
*Condensed	8-oz. serving	11.0
(Crosse & Blackwell)	6½-oz. serving	9.0
New England style:		
*(Campbell):		
Condensed:		
Made with milk	8-oz. serving	17.0
Made with water	8-oz. serving	11.0
Semi-condensed, *Soup For One:*		
Made with milk	11-oz. serving	23.0
Made with water	11-oz. serving	18.0
(Crosse & Blackwell)	6½-oz. serving	14.0
Ham'n potato (Hormel)	7½-oz. can	14.0
Consomme madrilene (Crosse & Blackwell)	6½-oz. serving	4.0
Crab (Crosse & Blackwell)	6½-oz. serving	8.0
Gazpacho (Crosse & Blackwell)	6½-oz. serving	1.0
Ham'n butter bean (Campbell) *Chunky*	10¾-oz. can	33.0
Lentil (Crosse & Blackwell) with ham	6½-oz. serving	13.0
*Meatball alphabet (Campbell) condensed	8-oz. serving	12.0
Minestrone:		
(Campbell):		
Chunky	19-oz. can	42.0
*Condensed	8-oz. serving	11.0
(Crosse & Blackwell)	6½-oz. serving	18.0
Mushroom:		
*(Campbell):		
Condensed:		
Cream of	8-oz. serving	9.0

Food and Description	*Measure or Quantity*	*Carbohydrates (grams)*
Golden	8-oz. serving	10.0
Semi-condensed,		
Soup For One,		
cream of, savory	11-oz. serving	10.0
(Crosse & Blackwell) cream of,		
bisque	6½-oz. serving	8.0
*(Rokeach) cream of		
Prepared with milk	10-oz. serving	20.0
Prepared with water	10-oz. serving	13.0
*Mushroom barley (Campbell)	8-oz. serving	12.0
*Noodle (Campbell) &		
ground beef	8-oz. serving	10.0
*Onion (Campbell):		
Regular	8-oz. serving	9.0
Cream of:		
Made with water	8-oz. serving	12.0
Made with water & milk	8-oz. serving	15.0
*Oyster stew (Campbell):		
Made with milk	8-oz. serving	10.0
Made with water	8-oz. serving	5.0
*Pea, green (Campbell)	8-oz. serving	25.0
Pea, split:		
(Campbell):		
Chunky, with ham	19-oz. can	58.0
*Condensed, with		
ham & bacon	8-oz. serving	24.0
(Grandma Brown's)	8-oz. serving	28.2
*Pepper pot (Campbell)	8-oz. serving	9.0
*Potato (Campbell) cream of:		
Made with water	8-oz. serving	11.0
Made with water & milk	8-oz. serving	14.0
Shav (Gold's)	8-oz. serving	2.1
Shrimp:		
*(Campbell) condensed,		
cream of:		
Made with milk	8-oz. serving	22.0
Made with water	8-oz. serving	8.0
(Crosse & Blackwell)	6½-oz. serving	7.0
Steak & potato (Campbell)		
Chunky	19-oz. can	42.0
Tomato:		
(Campbell):		
Condensed:		
Regular:		
Made with milk	8-oz. serving	22.0
Made with water	8-oz. serving	17.0

Food and Description	Measure or Quantity	Carbohydrates (grams)
& rice, old fashioned	8-oz. serving	22.0
Semi-condensed,		
Soup For One, Royale	11-oz. serving	35.0
*(Rokeach):		
Made with milk	10-oz. serving	27.0
Made with water	10-oz. serving	20.0
Turkey (Campbell) *Chunky*	18 ¾-oz. can	36.0
Vegetable:		
(Campbell):		
Chunky:		
Regular	19-oz. can	42.0
Beef, old fashioned	19-oz. can	18.0
*Condensed:		
Regular	8-oz. serving	12.0
Beef or vegetarian	10-oz. serving	8.0
*Semi-condensed,		
Soup For One, old world	11-oz. serving	18.0
*(Rokeach) vegetarian	10-oz. serving	15.0
Vichyssoise (Crosse & Blackwell)	6½-oz. serving	5.0
*Won ton (Campbell)	8-oz. serving	5.0
Canned, dietetic pack:		
Beef (Campbell) & mushroom, low sodium	10¾-oz. can	23.0
Chicken:		
(Campbell) low sodium:		
Chunky	7½-oz. can	14.0
Vegetable	10¾-oz. can	21.0
*(Dia-Mel) & noodle	8-oz. serving	11.0
Mushroom (Campbell) cream of, low sodium	7¼-oz. can	10.0
Pea, green (Campbell) low sodium	7½-oz. can	23.0
Pea, split (Campbell) low sodium	10¾-oz. can	35.0
Tomato (Campbell) low sodium:		
Regular	7¼-oz. can	24.0
With tomato pieces	10½-oz. can	32.0
Vegetable (Dia-Mel)	8-oz. serving	12.0
Frozen:		
*Barley & mushroom (Mother's Own)	8-oz. serving	8.0
Chowder, clam, New England style (Stouffer's)	8-oz. serving	19.0
Pea, split:		
*Mother's Own)	8-oz. serving	20.0
(Stouffer's)	8¼-oz. serving	27.0
Spinach (Stouffer's) cream of	8-oz. serving	17.0

Food and Description	*Measure or Quantity*	*Carbohydrates (grams)*
*Won ton (La Choy)	½ of 15-oz. pkg.	6.0
Mix, regular:		
Beef:		
**Carmel Kosher*	6 fl. oz.	1.8
*(Lipton) *Cup-A-Soup,* regular & noodle	6 fl. oz.	8.0
*(Weight Watchers) broth	6 fl. oz.	1.0
*Chicken:		
Carmel Kosher	6 fl. oz.	1.8
(Lipton):		
Cup-A-Broth	6 fl. oz.	4.0
Cup-A-Soup, & rice	6 fl. oz.	7.0
Country style, hearty	6 fl. oz.	10.0
Lots-A-Noodles	7 fl. oz.	23.0
*Noodle (Lipton):		
With chicken broth	8 fl. oz.	10.0
With chicken meat	8 fl. oz.	1.0
Giggle Noodle	8 fl. oz.	12.0
Ripple Noodle	8 fl. oz.	12.0
*Mushroom:		
Carmel Kosher	6 fl. oz.	2.0
(Lipton):		
Regular, beef	8 fl. oz.	7.0
Cup-A-Soup, cream of	6 fl. oz.	10.0
*Onion:		
Carmel Kosher	6 fl. oz.	2.4
(Lipton):		
Regular, beefy	8 fl. oz.	5.0
Regular, tomato	8 fl. oz.	15.0
Cup-A-Soup	6 fl. oz.	5.0
*Pea, green (Lipton) *Cup-A-Soup*	6 fl. oz.	16.0
*Tomato (Lipton) *Cup-A-Soup*	6 fl. oz.	17.0
*Vegetable:		
(Lipton):		
Regular, country	8 fl. oz.	14.0
Cup-A-Soup:		
Regular, spring	6 fl. oz.	7.0
Country style, harvest	6 fl. oz.	20.0
Lots-A-Noodles, garden	7 fl. oz.	23.0
(Southland) frozen	⅕ of 16-oz. pkg.	12.0
*Dietetic (Estee):		
Chicken, cream of	6½-oz. serving	8.0
Tomato, vegetable	6½-oz. serving	13.0
SOUTHERN COMFORT	1 fl. oz.	3.4
SOYBEAN CURD OR TOFU	2¾" × 1½" × 1" cake	2.9

Food and Description	Measure or Quantity	Carbohydrates (grams)
SPAGHETTI:		
Cooked:		
8–10 minutes, "Al Dente"	1 cup	43.9
14–20 minutes, tender	1 cup	32.2
Canned:		
(Franco-American):		
With meatballs in tomato sauce, *SpaghettiOs*	7⅜-oz. can	22.0
In meat sauce	7½-oz. can	26.0
With sliced franks in tomato sauce, *SpaghettiOs*	7⅜-oz. can	26.0
In tomato sauce with cheese	7⅜-oz. can	36.0
(Hormel) *Short Orders*, & meatballs in tomato sauce	7½-oz. can	26.0
(Libby's) & meatballs in tomato sauce	7½-oz. serving	27.5
Dietetic (Dia-Mel) & meatballs	8-oz. serving	24.0
Frozen:		
(Banquet)	8-oz. entree	35.0
(Green Giant) & meatballs in tomato sauce	10-oz. entree	53.9
(Morton)	8-oz. casserole	31.0
(Stouffer's) *Lean Cuisine*	11½-oz. pkg.	38.0
SPAGHETTI SAUCE, CANNED:		
Regular pack:		
Garden style (Ragu)	4-oz. serving	14.0
Marinara:		
(Prince)	4-oz. serving	12.4
(Ragu)	4-oz. serving	12.0
Meat or meat flavored:		
(Prego)	4-oz. serving	22.0
(Prince)	½ cup	11.0
(Ragu) regular	5-oz. serving	11.0
Meatless or plain:		
(Prego)	4-oz. serving	22.0
(Prince)	½ cup	11.4
(Ragu) Extra Thick & Zesty	4-oz. serving	15.0
Mushroom:		
(Hain)	4-oz. serving	14.3
(Prego)	4-oz. serving	22.0
(Prince)	4-oz. serving	11.3
(Ragu) regular	4-oz. serving	9.0
Dietetic pack (Featherweight)	⅔ cup	10.0
***SPAGHETTI SAUCE MIX:**		
(Durkee)	½ cup	10.4
(French's) with mushrooms	⅝ cup	13.0

Food and Description	*Measure or Quantity*	*Carbohydrates (grams)*
(Spatini)	½ cup	8.4
SPAM, luncheon meat (Hormel)	Any quantity	0.
SPECIAL K, cereal (Kellogg's)	1 cup	21.0
SPINACH:		
Fresh, whole leaves	½ cup	.7
Boiled	½ cup	2.8
Canned, regular pack (Sunshine) solids & liq.	½ cup	4.0
Frozen:		
(Birds Eye):		
Chopped or leaf	⅓ of pkg.	3.4
Creamed	⅓ of pkg.	4.9
(Green Giant):		
Creamed	½ cup	8.0
Harvest Fresh	½ cup	4.0
(McKenzie) chopped or cut	⅓ of pkg.	3.0
(Stouffer's) souffle	4-oz. serving	12.0
SQUASH, SUMMER:		
Yellow, boiled slices	½ cup	2.7
Zucchini, boiled slices	½ cup	1.9
Canned (Del Monte) zucchini, in tomato sauce	½ cup	8.0
Frozen:		
(Birds Eye) zucchini	⅓ of pkg.	3.3
(McKenzie) Crookneck	⅓ of pkg.	4.0
(Mrs. Paul's) zucchini sticks, breaded & fried	⅓ of pkg.	23.1
SQUASH, WINTER:		
Acorn, baked	½ cup	14.3
Hubbard, baked, mashed	½ cup	11.9
Frozen:		
(Birds Eye)	⅓ of pkg.	9.2
(Southland) butternut	4-oz. serving	16.0
STEAK & GREEN PEPPERS, frozen:		
(Green Giant)	9-oz. entree	32.0
(Swanson)	8½-oz. entree	12.0
STOCK BASE (French's) beef or chicken	1 tsp.	2.0
STRAWBERRY:		
Fresh, capped	½ cup	6.0
Frozen (Birds Eye):		
Halves, regular	⅓ of pkg.	34.9
Whole	¼ of pkg.	21.4
Whole, quick thaw	½ of pkg.	30.1
STRAWBERRY DRINK (Hi-C):		
Canned	6 fl. oz.	22.0

Food and Description	*Measure or Quantity*	*Carbohydrates (grams)*
*Mix	6 fl. oz.	17.0
STRAWBERRY NECTAR, canned		
(Libby's)	6 fl. oz.	14.0
STRAWBERRY PRESERVE OR JAM:		
Sweetened (Smucker's)	1 T.	13.5
Dietetic or low calorie:		
(Dia-Mel)	1 T.	0.
(Diet Delight)	1 T.	3.0
(Estee)	1 T.	1.6
(Louis Sherry)	1 T.	0.
STUFFING MIX:		
*Chicken, *Stove Top*	½ cup	20.2
*Cornbread, *Stove Top*	½ cup	21.6
Cube or herb seasoned		
(Pepperidge Farm)	1 oz.	22.0
*Pork, *Stove Top*	½ cup	20.3
White bread (Mrs. Cubbison's)	1 oz.	20.5
SUCCOTASH:		
Canned:		
(Libby's) cream style	½ cup	22.8
(Stokely-Van Camp)	½ cup	17.5
Frozen (Birds Eye)	⅓ of pkg.	20.7
SUGAR:		
Brown	1 T.	12.5
Confectioners'	1 T.	7.7
Granulated	1 T.	11.9
Maple	1¾" × 1¼" × ½" piece	27.0
SUGAR CORN POPS, cereal		
(Kellogg's)	1 cup	26.0
SUGAR CRISP, cereal (Post)	⅞ cup	25.6
SUGAR PUFFS, cereal		
(Malt-O-Meal)	⅞ cup	26.0
SUGAR SMACKS, cereal (Kellogg's)	¾ cup	25.0
SUGAR SUBSTITUTE:		
(Estee)	1 tsp.	3.0
(Featherweight)	3 drops	0.
Sprinkle Sweet (Pillsbury)	1 tsp.	.5
Sweet'n-it (Dia-Mel) liquid	5 drops	0.
SUNFLOWER SEED (Fisher)		
In hull, roasted, salted	1 oz.	3.0
Hulled, dry or oil roasted, salted	1 oz.	5.6
SUZY Q (Hostess):		
Banana	1 piece	38.0
Chocolate	1 piece	37.0
SWEETBREADS	Any quantity	0.

Food and Description	*Measure or Quantity*	*Carbohydrates (grams)*
SWEET POTATO:		
Baked, peeled	5″ × 1″ potato	35.8
Canned, heavy syrup	4-oz. serving	31.2
Frozen (Stouffer's) with apple	5-oz. serving	31.0
SWEET & SOUR PORK, frozen (La Choy)	12-oz. entree	64.0
SWISS STEAK, frozen (Swanson) *TV Brand*	10-oz. dinner	37.0
SWORDFISH, broiled	Any quantity	0.
SYRUP (See also TOPPING):		
Regular:		
Apricot (Smucker's)	1 T.	13.0
Blackberry (Smucker's)	1 T.	13.0
Chocolate or chocolate-flavored:		
Bosco	1 T.	13.3
(Hershey's)	1 T.	11.7
Corn, *Karo,* dark or light	1 T.	14.6
Maple, *Karo,* imitation	1 T.	14.2
Pancake or waffle:		
(Aunt Jemima)	1 T.	13.1
Golden Griddle	1 T.	13.3
Karo	1 T.	14.4
Log Cabin, regular or buttered	1 T.	14.0
Mrs. Butterworth's	1 T.	13.0
Strawberry (Smucker's)	1 T.	13.0
Dietetic or low calorie:		
Blueberry (Featherweight)	1 T.	3.0
Chocolate or chocolate-flavored (Diet Delight)	1 T.	2.0
Coffee (No-Cal)	1 T.	1.2
Cola (No-Cal)	1 T.	Tr.
Maple (S&W) *Nutradiet*	1 T.	3.0
Pancake or waffle:		
(Aunt Jemima)	1 T.	7.3
(Dia-Mel)	1 T.	Tr.
(Diet Delight)	1 T.	4.0
(Featherweight)	1 T.	3.0
(S&W) *Nutradiet*	1 T.	1.0

T

Food and Description	Measure or Quantity	Carbohydrates (grams)
TACO:		
*(Ortega)	1 taco	15.0
*Mix (Durkee)	½ cup	3.8
Shell (Ortega)	1 shell	7.7
TAMALE, frozen (Hormel) beef	1 tamale	13.0
TANG:		
Grape	6 fl. oz.	23.2
Orange	6 fl. oz.	21.8
TANGERINE OR MANDARIN ORANGE:		
Fresh (Sunkist)	1 large tangerine	10.0
Canned, solids & liq.:		
Regular pack (Del Monte)	5½-oz. serving	25.0
Dietetic pack:		
(Diet Delight) juice pack	½ cup	13.0
(Featherweight) water pack	½ cup	8.0
(S&W) *Nutradiet*	½ cup	7.0
TANGERINE DRINK, canned (Hi-C)	6 fl. oz.	23.0
***TANGERINE JUICE,** frozen (Minute Maid)	6 fl. oz.	20.8
TAPIOCA, dry, *Minute,* quick cooking	1 T.	7.9
TAQUITO, frozen (Van de Kamp's) beef	8-oz. serving	47.0
TARRAGON (French's)	1 tsp.	.7
TASTEEOS, cereal (Ralston Purina)	1 ¼ cups	22.0
***TEA:**		
Bag:		
(Lipton):		
Plain	1 cup	0.
Flavored	1cup	Tr.
Herbal:		
Almond pleasure or		

Food and Description	*Measure or Quantity*	*Carbohydrates (grams)*
cinnamon apple	1 cup	Tr.
Quietly chamomile or		
toasty spice	1 cup	1.0
(Sahadi) spearmint	1 cup	Tr.
Instant (Nestea)	8 fl. oz.	0.
TEA MIX, ICED:		
*(Lipton) lemon & sugar flavored	1 cup	16.0
**Nestea,* lemon-flavored	1 cup	1.0
*Dietetic, *Crystal Light*	8 fl. oz.	.2
TEQUILA SUNRISE COCKTAIL		
(Mr. Boston) 12 ½% alcohol	3 fl. oz.	14.4
TERIYAKI, frozen (Stouffer's)	10-oz. serving	26.0
***TEXTURED VEGETABLE**		
PROTEIN, *Morningstar Farms:*		
Breakfast link	1 link	1.3
Breakfast patties	1 patty	3.5
Breakfast strips	1 strip	.7
Grillers	1 patty	6.0
THURINGER:		
(Eckrich)	1-oz. serving	0.
(Hormel):		
Buffet or tangy, chub	1-oz. serving	0.
Old Smokehouse	1-oz. serving	1.0
(Louis Rich) turkey	1-oz. serving	Tr.
(Oscar Mayer)	.8-oz. slice	.7
TIGER TAILS (Hostess)	2 ¼-oz. piece	38.0
TOASTER CAKE OR PASTRY:		
Pop-Tarts (Kellogg's):		
Regular:		
Blueberry or cherry	1 pastry	36.0
Strawberry	1 pastry	37.0
Frosted:		
Blueberry or strawberry	1 pastry	38.0
Brown sugar cinnamon	1 pastry	34.0
Chocolate-vanilla creme	1 pastry	37.0
Toaster Strudel (Pillsbury)	1 piece	27.0
Toast-R-Cake (Thomas'):		
Blueberry	1 piece	17.7
Bran	1 piece	18.5
Corn	1 piece	17.4
TOASTIES, cereal (Post)	1 ¼ cups	24.4
TOMATO:		
Cherry, whole	4 pieces	3.2
Regular, whole	1 med. tomato	7.0
Canned, regular pack, solids & liq.:		
(Contadina) sliced, baby	½ cup	10.0

Food and Description	*Measure or Quantity*	*Carbohydrates (grams)*
(Del Monte) stewed or wedges	4 oz.	8.0
(Stokely-Van Camp) stewed	½ cup	7.5
Canned, dietetic pack, solids & liq.:		
(Del Monte) No Salt Added	½ cup	8.0
(Diet Delight)	½ cup	5.0
(Featherweight)	½ cup	4.0
TOMATO JUICE, CANNED:		
Regular pack:		
(Campbell; Libby's)	6-fl.-oz. can	8.0
(Del Monte)	6-fl.-oz. can	7.4
Musselman's	6-fl.-oz. can	7.0
Dietetic pack (Diet Delight; Featherweight)	6 fl. oz.	7.0
TOMATO JUICE COCKTAIL, canned:		
(Ocean Spray) *Firehouse Jubilee*	6 fl. oz.	9.1
Snap-E-Tom	6 fl. oz.	7.0
TOMATO PASTE, canned:		
Regular pack:		
(Contadina) Italian	6-oz. serving	36.0
(Del Monte) regular or No Salt Added	6-oz. can	34.0
Dietetic (Featherweight) low sodium	6-oz. can	35.0
TOMATO & PEPPER, HOT CHILI (Ortega) Jalapeno	1-oz. serving	1.1
TOMATO, PICKLED (Claussen) green	1 piece	1.1
TOMATO PUREE, canned:		
Regular (Contadina) heavy	½ cup	11.0
Dietetic (Featherweight)	½ cup	10.0
TOMATO SAUICE, canned:		
(Contadina) regular	½ cup	9.0
(Del Monte) regular or No Salt Added	½ cup	8.0
(Hunt's) with cheese	4-oz. serving	10.0
TOM COLLINS (Mr. Boston) 12½% alcohol	3 fl. oz.	10.8
TONGUE, beef, braised	4-oz. serving	.5
TOPPING:		
Regular:		
Butterscotch (Smucker's)	1 T.	16.5
Caramel (Smucker's)	1 T.	16.5
Chocolate fudge (Hershey's)	1 T.	7.3
Pecans in syrup (Smucker's)	1 T.	14.0
Pineapple (Smucker's)	1 T.	16.0
Dietetic, chocolate (Diet Delight)	1 T.	3.6

Food and Description	*Measure or Quantity*	*Carbohydrates (grams)*
TOPPING, WHIPPED:		
Regular:		
Cool Whip (Birds Eye) dairy	1 T.	1.2
Dover Farms, dairy	1 T.	1.2
Lucky Whip, aerosol	1 T.	.5
Whip Topping (Rich's)	¼ oz.	1.2
Dietetic (Featherweight)	1 T.	.5
*Mix:		
Regular, *Dream Whip*	1 T.	.9
Dietetic, (D-Zerta)	1 T.	.2
TOP RAMEN, beef (Nissin Foods)	3-oz. serving	50.5
TORTILLA (Amigos)	6″ × ⅛″ tortilla	19.7
TOSTADA, frozen (Van de Kamp's)	8½-oz. serving	37.0
TOSTADA SHELL (Ortega)	1 shell	6.0
TOTAL, cereal	1 cup	23.0
TRIPE, canned (Libby's)	6-oz. serving	1.1
TRIPLE SEC LIQUEUR (Mr. Boston)	1 fl. oz.	8.5
TRIX, cereal (General Mills)	1 cup	25.0
TUNA	Any quantity	0.
****TUNA HELPER*** (General Mills):		
Country dumplings	⅕ of pkg.	31.0
Noodles/cheese	⅕ of pkg.	28.0
TUNA NOODLE CASSEROLE, frozen (Stouffer's)	5 ¾-oz. serving	18.0
TUNA PIE, frozen:		
(Banquet)	8-oz. pie	48.0
(Morton)	8-oz. pie	36.0
TURKEY:		
Barbecued (Louis Rich) breast, half	1 oz.	0.
Canned:		
(Hormel) chunk	6¾-oz. serving	Tr.
(Swanson) chunk	2½-oz. serving	0.
Packaged:		
(Hormel) breast	1 slice	0.
(Louis Rich):		
Turkey bologna	1-oz. slice	1.0
Turkey cotto salami	1-oz. slice	Tr.
Turkey ham, chopped	1-oz. slice	Tr.
Turkey pastrami	1-oz. slice	Tr.
(Oscar Mayer) breast	¾-oz. slice	0.
Roasted	Any quantity	0.
Smoked (Louis Rich):		
Drumsticks	1 oz. (without bone)	Tr.
Wing drumettes	1 oz.	

Food and Description	*Measure or Quantity*	*Carbohydrates (grams)*
	(without bone)	Tr.
TURKEY DINNER OR ENTREE, FROZEN:		
(Banquet):		
American Favorites	11-oz. dinner	41.0
Extra Helping	19-oz. dinner	98.0
(Green Giant)	9-oz. entree	34.0
(Morton) regular	5-oz. entree	5.0
(Swanson):		
Regular, with gravy & dressing	9¼-oz. entree	25.0
Hungry Man	18¾-oz. dinner	70.0
TV Brand	11½-oz. dinner	40.0
(Weight Watchers) sliced, 3-compartment	15¼-oz. meal	32.0
TURKEY PIE, frozen:		
(Banquet):		
Regular	8-oz. pie	32.0
Supreme	8-oz. pie	41.0
(Morton)	8-oz. pie	31.0
(Stouffer's)	10-oz. pie	35.0
(Swanson) regular	8-oz. pie	39.0
TURKEY SALAD, canned (Carnation)	2-oz. serving	3.1
TURKEY TETRAZINI, frozen:		
(Stouffer's)	6-oz. serving	17.0
(Weight Watchers)	10-oz. pkg.	28.0
TURMERIC (French's)	1 tsp.	1.3
TURNIP GREENS, canned (Sunshine) chopped, solids & liq.	½ cup	2.5
TURNOVER:		
Frozen (Pepperidge Farm):		
Apple	1 turnover	35.0
Blueberry or cherry	1 turnover	32.0
Peach	1 turnover	34.0
Refrigerated (Pillsbury):		
Apple or blueberry	1 turnover	22.0
Cherry	1 turnover	24.0
TWINKIE (Hostess):		
Regular	1 piece	26.0
Devil's food	1 piece	24.7

V

Food and Description	*Measure or Quantity*	*Carbohydrates (grams)*
VALPOLICELLA WINE (Antinori)	3 fl. oz.	6.3
VANDERMINT, liqueur	1 fl. oz.	10.2
VEAL	Any quantity	0.
VEAL DINNER, FROZEN:		
(Banquet) parmigiana	11-oz. dinner	43.0
(Morton) regular	5-oz. pkg.	14.0
(Swanson) parmigiana:		
Hungry Man	20½-oz. dinner	61.0
TV Brand	12 ¼-oz. dinner	46.0
(Weight Watchers) parmigiana, 2-compartment	9-oz. meal	23.0
VEAL STEAK, FROZEN (Hormel):		
Regular	4-oz. serving	2.0
Breaded	4-oz. serving	13.0
VEGETABLE BOUILLON (Herb-Ox):		
Cube	1 cube	.6
Packet	1 packet	2.2
VEGETABLE JUICE COCKTAIL:		
Regular, *V-8*	6 fl. oz.	8.0
Dietetic:		
(S&W) *Nutradiet*, low sodium	6 fl. oz.	8.0
V-8, low sodium	6 fl. oz.	9.0
VEGETABLES, MIXED:		
Canned, regular pack:		
(Del Monte) solids & liq.	½ cup	2.0
(La Choy) drained:		
Chinese	⅓ of 14-oz. pkg.	2.0
Chop Suey	½ cup	2.0
(Libby's) solids & liq.	½ cup	9.8
Canned, dietetic pack (Featherweight)	½ cup	8.0
Frozen:		
(Birds Eye):		

Food and Description	*Measure or Quantity*	*Carbohydrates (grams)*
Regular:		
Broccoli, cauliflower & carrots in butter sauce	⅓ of pkg.	5.7
Carrots, peas & onions, deluxe	⅓ of pkg.	10.0
Mixed, with onion sauce	⅓ of pkg.	11.6
Pea & pearl onion	⅓ of pkg.	13.5
Farm Fresh:		
Broccoli, cauliflower & carrot strips	⅕ of pkg.	5.3
Brussels sprouts, cauliflower & carrots	⅕ of pkg.	6.5
International Style:		
Chinese style	⅓ of pkg.	8.4
Mexican style	⅓ of pkg.	16.1
Stir Fry:		
Chinese style	⅓ of pkg.	6.9
Japanese style	⅓ of pkg.	5.9
(Green Giant):		
Regular:		
Broccoli, cauliflower & carrots in cheese sauce	½ cup	8.0
Mixed, polybag	½ cup	10.0
Harvest Fresh	½ cup	13.0
Harvest Get Togethers:		
Broccoli-cauliflower medley	½ cup	10.0
Broccoli fanfare	½ cup	14.0
Japanese style	½ cup	8.0
(La Choy):		
Chinese	3.3-oz. serving	5.0
Japanese	3.3-oz. serving	5.8
(Le Sueur) peas, onions & carrots in butter sauce	½ cup	11.0
(Southland):		
California blend	⅕ of 16-oz. pkg.	7.0
Stew	4 oz.	14.0
VEGETABLES IN PASTRY, FROZEN		
(Pepperidge Farm):		
Asparagus with mornay sauce or broccoli with cheese	3 ¾ oz.	18.0
Cauliflower & cheese sauce	3 ¾ oz.	20.0
Spinach almondine	3 ¾ oz.	19.0
Zucchini provencal	3 ¾ oz.	21.0
VEGETABLE STEW, canned		
Dinty Moore (Hormel)	8-oz. serving	20.0

Food and Description	Measure or Quantity	Carbohydrates (grams)
"VEGETARIAN FOODS":		
Canned or dry:		
Chicken, fried (Loma Linda) with gravy	1½-oz. piece	3.4
Chili (Worthington)	½ can	13.2
Choplet (Worthington)	1 slice	1.7
Dinner cuts (Loma Linda)	1 piece	1.6
Franks, big (Loma Linda)	1.9-oz. frank	4.1
Franks, sizzle (Loma Linda)	2.2-oz. frank	4.6
FriChik (Worthington)	1 piece	2.5
Granburger (Worthington)	1 oz.	5.8
Little links (Loma Linda) drained	.8-oz. link	1.3
Non-meatballs (Worthington)	1 meatball	1.9
Nuteena (Loma Linda)	½" slice	7.6
Proteena (Loma Linda)	½" slice	6.5
Sandwich spread:		
(Loma Linda)	1 T.	1.7
(Worthington)	2½ oz.	2.0
Savorex (Loma Linda)	1 T.	2.0
Soyalac (Loma Linda):		
Concentrate, liquid	1 cup	33.8
Ready to use	1 cup	15.9
Soyameat (Worthington):		
Beef, sliced	1 slice	2.6
Chicken, diced	1 oz.	1.4
Salisbury steak	1 slice	2.0
Soyamel, any kind (Worthington)	1 oz.	12.2
Stew pack (Loma Linda) drained	1 piece	.6
Super links (Worthington)	1 link	3.7
Swiss steak with gravy (Loma Linda)	1 steak	8.9
Tender bits (Loma Linda) drained	1 piece	1.1
Vegelona (Loma Linda)	½" slice	7.0
Vega-links (Worthington)	1 link	2.8
Wheat protein	4 oz.	10.0
Worthington 209	1 slice	2.2
Frozen:		
Beef-like slices (Worthington)	1 slice	2.0
Beef pie (Worthington)	1 pie	41.8
Bologna (Loma Linda)	1 oz.	1.2
Chicken (Loma Linda)	1 slice	1.5
Chicken, fried (Loma Linda)	2-oz. serving	3.6
Chicken pie (Worthington)	1 pie	37.5
Chic-Ketts (Worthington)	1 oz.	2.2

Food and Description	*Measure or Quantity*	*Carbohydrates (grams)*
Corned beef, loaf or sliced (Worthington)	2½ oz.	6.0
FriPats (Worthington)	1 pat	5.2
Meatballs (Loma Linda)	1 meatball	2.2
Prosage (Worthington)	1 link	1.5
Roast beef (Loma Linda)	1 oz.	1.3
Sausage, breakfast (Loma Linda)	⅓" slice	1.4
Smoked beef, roll (Worthington)	2½ oz.	1.0
Turkey (Loma Linda)	1 oz.	1.6
Wham, roll (Worthington)	2½ oz.	4.0
VERMOUTH:		
Dry & extra dry (Lejon)	1 fl. oz.	2.2
Sweet (Lejon; Taylor)	1 fl. oz.	3.8
VICHY WATER (Schweppes)	Any quantity	0.
VIENNA SAUSAGE (See SAUSAGE, Vienna)		
VINEGAR	1 T.	.8

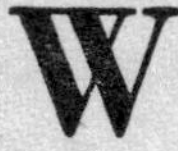

Food and Description	Measure or Quantity	Carbohydrates (grams)
WAFFELOS, cereal (Ralston Purina)	1 cup	25.0
WAFFLE, frozen:		
(Aunt Jemima) jumbo	1 waffle	14.5
(Eggo):		
Apple cinnamon	1 waffle	20.0
Home style or blueberry	1 waffle	16.0
WALNUT (Fisher)	½ cup	8.8
WATER CHESTNUT, canned		
(La Choy) drained	¼ of 8-oz. can	4.0
WATERCRESS, trimmed	½ cup	.5
WATERMELON:		
Wedge	4″ × 8″ wedge	27.3
Diced	½ cup	5.1
WELSH RAREBIT:		
Home recipe	1 cup	14.6
Frozen:		
(Green Giant)	5-oz. serving	11.4
(Stouffer's)	5-oz. serving	17.0
WESTERN DINNER, frozen:		
(Banquet)	11-oz. dinner	43.0
(Morton)	11.8-oz. dinner	32.0
(Swanson):		
Hungry Man	17 ¾-oz. dinner	73.0
TV Brand	11 ¾-oz. dinner	45.0
WHEATENA, cereal	¼ cup	22.5
WHEAT FLAKES CEREAL		
(Featherweight)	1 ¼ cups	23.0
WHEAT GERM, RAW (Elam's)	1 T.	3.2
WHEAT GERM CEREAL		
(Kretschmer):		
Regular	¼ cup	8.8
Brown sugar & honey	¼ cup	17.0
WHEAT HEARTS, cereal		
(General Mills)	1 oz.	21.0

Food and Description	*Measure or Quantity*	*Carbohydrates (grams)*
WHEATIES, cereal	1 cup	23.0
WHEAT & OATMEAL CEREAL,		
hot (Elam's)	1 oz.	18.8
WHISKEY SOUR COCKTAIL		
(Mr. Boston)	3 fl. oz.	14.4
WHITE CASTLE:		
Bun	.8-oz. bun	12.4
Cheeseburger (meat & cheese only)	1.54-oz. serving	5.2
Fish sandwich (fish only, without tartar sauce & bun)	1.5-oz. serving	7.8
French fries	2.6-oz. serving	15.1
Hamburger (meat only, no bun)	1.2-oz. serving	5.2
WHITEFISH, LAKE:		
Baked, stuffed	4 oz.	6.6
Smoked	4 oz.	0.
WILD BERRY DRINK,		
canned (Hi-C)	6 fl. oz.	22.0
WINCHELL'S DONUT HOUSE:		
Buttermilk, old fashioned	2-oz. piece	56.0
Cake, devil's food, iced	2-oz. piece	54.0
Raised apple fritter	4½-oz. piece	48.8
Raised, glazed	1 ¾-oz. piece	48.5
WINE, COOKING (Regina):		
Burgundy or sauterne	¼ cup	Tr.
Sherry	¼ cup	5.0

Y

Food and Description	Measure or Quantity	Carbohydrates (grams)
YEAST, BAKER'S (Fleischmann's):		
Dry, active	¼ oz.	3.0
Fresh & household, active	.6-oz. cake	2.0
YOGURT:		
Regular:		
Plain:		
(Bison)	8-oz. container	16.8
(Colombo):		
Regular	8-oz. container	13.0
Natural Lite	8-oz. container	17.0
(Dannon)	8-oz. container	15.0
(Friendship)	8-oz. container	15.0
Yoplait	6-oz. container	14.0
Plain with honey, *Yoplait, Custard Style*	6-oz. container	23.0
Apple:		
(Colombo) spiced	8-oz. container	39.0
(Dannon) Dutch	8-oz. container	49.0
Melange	6-oz. container	31.0
Yoplait	6-oz. container	32.0
Apple-cinnamon, *Yoplait, Breakfast Yogurt*	6-oz. container	40.0
Apricot (Bison)	8-oz. container	45.9
Banana (Dannon)	8-oz. container	49.0
Banana-strawberry (Colombo)	8-oz. container	38.0
Berry (New Country) mixed	8-oz. container	40.0
Blueberry:		
(Bison):		
Regular	8-oz. container	45.9
Light	6-oz. container	28.1
(Colombo)	8-oz. container	38.0
(Dannon)	8-oz. container	49.0
(Friendship)	8-oz. container	44.0
Melange	6-oz. container	31.0

Food and Description	*Measure or Quantity*	*Carbohydrates (grams)*
(New Country) supreme	8-oz. container	40.0
(Riche)	6-oz. container	33.0
(Sweet'n Low)	8-oz. container	33.0
Yoplait	6-oz. container	32.0
Boysenberry:		
(Bison)	8-oz. container	45.9
(Dannon)	8-oz. container	49.0
(Sweet'n Low)	8-oz. container	33.0
Cherry:		
(Colombo) black	8-oz. container	34.0
(Dannon)	8-oz. container	49.0
(Riche)	6-oz. container	33.0
(Sweet'n Low)	8-oz. container	33.0
Yoplait	6-oz. container	32.0
Cherry-vanilla (Colombo)	8-oz. container	40.0
Citrus, *Yoplait, Breakfast Yogurt*	6-oz. container	43.0
Coffee (Colombo)	8-oz. container	29.0
Date-walnut-raisin (Bison)	8-oz. container	45.9
Fruit crunch (New Country)	8-oz. container	40.0
Granola strawberry (Colombo)	8-oz. container	40.0
Guava (Colombo)	8-oz. container	40.0
Hawaiian salad (New Country)	8-oz. container	40.0
Honey vanilla (Colombo)	8-oz. container	30.0
Lemon:		
(Dannon)	8-oz. container	32.0
(Sweet'n Low)	8-oz. container	33.0
Yoplait:		
Regular	6-oz. container	32.0
Custard Style	6-oz. container	30.0
Orange, *Yoplait*	6-oz. container	32.0
Orange supreme (New Country)	8-oz. container	40.0
Orchard, *Yoplait, Breakfast Yogurt*	6-oz. container	40.0
Peach:		
(Bison)	8-oz. container	45.9
(Dannon)	8-oz. container	49.0
(Friendship)	8-oz. container	44.0
(Meadow Gold)	8-oz. container	48.0
(Riche)	6-oz. container	33.0
(Sweet'N Low)	8-oz. container	33.0
Peach melba (Colombo)	8-oz. container	37.0
Pina colada:		
(Colombo)	8-oz. container	40.0
(Dannon)	8-oz. container	49.0
(Friendship)	8-oz. container	44.0

Food and Description	*Measure or Quantity*	*Carbohydrates (grams)*
Pineapple:		
(Bison) light	6-oz. container	28.1
Melange	6-oz. container	31.0
Raspberry:		
(Colombo)	8-oz. container	39.0
(Dannon) red	8-oz. container	49.0
(Friendship)	8-oz. container	44.0
Melange	6-oz. container	31.0
(Riche)	6-oz. container	33.0
(Sweet'N Low)	8-oz. container	33.0
Yoplait:		
Regular	6-oz. container	32.0
Custard Style	6-oz. container	30.0
Strawberry:		
(Bison) light	6-oz. container	28.1
(Colombo)	8-oz. container	36.0
(Dannon)	8-oz. container	49.0
(Friendship)	8-oz. container	49.0
(Meadow Gold)	8-oz. container	49.0
(Sweet'N Low)	8-oz. container	33.0
Yoplait	6-oz. container	32.0
Strawberry-banana (Riché)	6-oz. container	33.0
Strawberry colada (Colombo)	8-oz. container	36.0
Tropical fruit (Sweet'N Low)	8-oz. container	33.0
Vanilla:		
(Dannon)	8-oz. container	32.0
(New Country) french ripple	8-oz. container	40.0
Yoplait, Custard Style	6-oz. container	30.0
Frozen, hard:		
Banana, *Danny-in-a-Cup*	8-oz. cup	42.0
Boysenberry, *Danny-on-a-Stick,* carob coated	2½-fl.-oz. bar	15.0
Boysenberry swirl (Bison)	¼ of 16-oz. container	24.0
Cherry vanilla (Bison)	¼ of 16-oz. container	24.0
Chocolate:		
(Bison)	¼ of 16-oz. container	24.0
(Colombo) bar, chocolate coated	1 bar	17.0
(Dannon):		
Danny-in-a-Cup	8-fl.-oz. cup	32.0
Danny-on-a-Stick, chocolate coated	2 ½-fl.-oz. bar	12.0
Chocolate chip (Bison)	¼ of 16-oz.	

Food and Description	*Measure or Quantity*	*Carbohydrates (grams)*
	container	24.0
Chocolate chocolate chip (Colombo)	4-oz. serving	28.0
Mocha (Colombo) bar	1 bar	14.0
Pina colada:		
(Colombo)	4-oz. serving	20.0
(Dannon):		
Danny-in-a-Cup	8-oz. cup	44.0
Danny-on-a-Stick	2 ½-fl.-oz. bar	14.0
Raspberry, red (Dannon):		
Danny-on-a-Stick, chocolate coated	2½-fl.-oz. bar	15.0
Danny-in-a-Cup	8-oz. container	42.0
Raspberry swirl (Bison)	¼ of 16-oz. container	24.0
Strawberry:		
(Bison)	¼ of 16-oz. container	24.0
(Colombo):		
Regular	4-oz. serving	20.0
Bar	1 bar	14.0
(Dannon) *Danny-in-a-Cup*	8 fl. oz.	42.0
Vanilla:		
(Bison)	¼ of 16-oz. container	24.0
(Colombo):		
Regular	4-oz. serving	20.0
Bar, chocolate coated	1 bar	17.0
(Dannon):		
Danny-in-a-Cup	8 fl. oz.	33.0
Danny-on-a-Stick	2½-fl.-oz. bar	11.0
Frozen, soft:		
(Colombo)	6-fl.-oz. serving	24.0
(Dannon) *Danny-Yo*	3½-fl.-oz. serving	21.0

Z

Food and Description	*Measure or Quantity*	*Carbohydrates (grams)*
ZINFANDEL WINE (Inglenook)		
Vintage	3 fl. oz.	.3
ZITI, FROZEN (Weight Watchers)	11 ¼-oz. serving	30.0
ZWEIBACK (Gerber; Nabisco)	1 piece	5.0

Staying Healthy with SIGNET Books

(0451)

☐ **MEGA-NUTRITION by Richard A Kunin. M.D.** Devised by a preeminent medical authority, this is the diet-plus-vitamins program to prevent disease, treat illness, promote good health... "I hope that everyone will read *Mega-Nutrition* and benefit from it."—Linus Pauling, Nobel Prize-winning scientist (129598—$3.95)*

☐ **BEAUTIFUL BODY BUILDING: Weight Training for Women for Fitness, Strength and Good Looks by Deirdre S. Lakein.** An expert provides programs and suggestions for using weight training to improve fitness, strength and appearance, offers advice on selecting a health club as well as setting up a home gym. Includes instructions for exercising with dumbbells and barbells and with new equipment such as the Nautilus and Universal machines. Photographs, Index included. (129865—$2.95)*

☐ **JOGGING, AEROBICS AND DIET: One Is Not Enough—You Need All Three by Roy Ald, with a Foreword by M. Thomas Woodall, Ph.D.** A personalized prescription for health, vitality, and general well-being based on a revolutionary new theory of exercise. (119770—$2.50)

☐ **YOGA FOR AMERICANS By Indra Devi.** A complete six-week home course in the widely recognized science that offers its practitioners a vital and confident approach to the pressures and tensions of modern living. (098692—$2.25)

☐ **EATING IS OKAY! A Radical Approach to Weight Loss: The Behavioral Control Diet by Henry A. Jordon, M.D., Leonard S. Levitz, Ph.D., and Gordon M. Kimbrell, Ph.D.** You can get thin and stay thin by changing your life style—say the doctors of this phenomenally successful Behavioral Weight Control Clinic. (127315—$2.50)*

*Prices slightly higher in Canada

Buy them at your local bookstore or use this convenient coupon for ordering.

**NEW AMERICAN LIBRARY,
P.O. Box 999, Bergenfield, New Jersey 07621**

Please send me the books I have checked above. I am enclosing $______ (please add $1.00 to this order to cover postage and handling). Send check or money order—no cash or C.O.D.'s. Prices and numbers are subject to change without notice.

Name____________________

Address____________________

City__________ State__________ Zip Code__________

**Allow 4-6 weeks for delivery.
This offer is subject to withdrawal without notice.**